Uric Acid in Chronic Kidney Disease

Contributions to Nephrology

Vol. 192

Series Editor

Claudio Ronco Vicenza

Uric Acid in Chronic Kidney Disease

Volume Editors

Alejandro Treviño-Becerra Mexico City
Kunitoshi Iseki Okinawa

18 figures, 3 in color, and 11 tables, 2018

KARGER Basel · Freiburg · Paris · London · New York · Chennai · New Delhi · Bangkok · Beijing · Shanghai · Tokyo · Kuala Lumpur · Singapore · Sydney

Contributions to Nephrology
(Founded 1975 by Geoffrey M. Berlyne)

Alejandro Treviño-Becerra
Uremic and Dialysis Clinic
Tuxpan 16-104 Col. Roma
06760 México City (México)

Kunitoshi Iseki
Clinical Research Support Center
Tomishiro Central Hospital
25 Ueta, Tomigusuku
Okinawa 901-0243 (Japan)

Library of Congress Cataloging-in-Publication Data

Title: Uric acid in chronic kidney disease / volume editors, Alejandro Treviño-Becerra, Kunitoshi Iseki.
Other titles: Contributions to nephrology ; v. 192. 0302-5144
Description: Basel ; New York : Karger, [2018] | Series: Contributions to nephrology, ISSN 0302-5144 ; vol. 192 | Includes bibliographical references and indexes.
Identifiers: LCCN 2017057195| ISBN 9783318062502 (hard cover : alk. paper) | ISBN 9783318062519 (e-ISBN)
Subjects: | MESH: Renal Insufficiency, Chronic | Hyperuricemia | Uric Acid--blood | Diabetic Nephropathies | Gout
Classification: LCC RC632.H89 | NLM WJ 342 | DDC 616.3/99--dc23 LC record available at https://lccn.loc.gov/2017057195

www.karger.com
Printed on acid-free and non-aging paper (ISO 9706)
ISSN 0302–5144
e-ISSN 1662–2782
ISBN 978–3–318–06250–2
e-ISBN 978–3–318–06251–9

Contents

Foreword

I am very grateful to the Editorial Division of Karger Publishers for choosing to publish this book in the prestigious *Contributions to Nephrology* series. This publication aims to achieve the widespread dissemination of recent knowledge acquired in the field of nephrology, especially in light of the cancellation of the International Satellite Symposium on Uric Acid in Chronic Renal Disease that was to be held in April 2017.

In 1979, I had the opportunity to publish the 17th volume of this series, entitled *Today's Art of Peritoneal Dialysis*, following the First International Symposium on Peritoneal Dialysis held in Chapala, Jalisco, Mexico in 1978. Dr. Fred S.T. Boen, who sadly passed away in 2017, was the coeditor. That publication contributed much to the global objective of improving processes related to the development of peritoneal dialysis. I sincerely hope that this latest edition will also aid the enhancement of current knowledge on this subject.

In 1979 I was just beginning my career in the field of nephrology. Now, almost 40 years later, I consider my involvement in publishing volume 192 of the series as a significant milestone in my career. I would like to express my gratitude to all the authors, especially Prof. Kunitoshi Iseki, who worked diligently to procure several chapters of this volume from other outstanding colleagues in Asia and a friendly recognition of Prof. Claudio Ronco for his interest in this field of the medicine and his enthusiastic support of this publication.

Dr. Alejandro Treviño-Becerra

Introduction

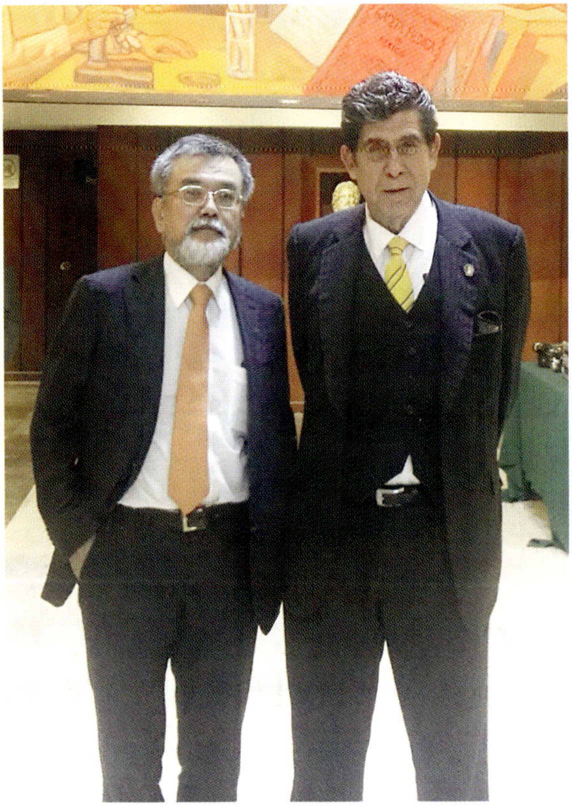

The idea of conducting a scientific meeting devoted to uric acid and chronic renal diseases was developed during the 8th and 9th Congresses of Uremia Toxicity and Research held in Okinawa, Japan, and Guadalajara, Mexico. In April 2016, during the 17th international Congress of Nutrition and Metabolism of Renal Diseases in Okinawa, a committee was formed with Prof. Kunitoshi Iseki and myself as the chairmen. Faculty members were invited to plan an interesting program, the products of which are published in this book.

Unfortunately, for various reasons, the symposium had to be cancelled just a few weeks before its scheduled event. However, the authors decided to remain true to their commitment to make possible the publication of their work, for which I am grateful to them all.

More than 30 years ago, in order to become a member of the National Academy of Medicine in Mexico, I presented my work relating to studies performed on 23 patients with uric acid reduction. This was achieved through an isocaloric, low-protein, and purine diet, as well as high doses of allopurinol, resulting in a blood urea reduction of 15–20% and a slightly increased creatinine clearance of up to 15–20%. Since then, we have routinely used the findings of those studies to acquire the benefits of low blood uric acid in our patients, which from the initiation of treatment provides relief through the reduction of some of their symptoms, mainly related to the gastrointestinal system. This in turn allows them to feel better and more able to cope with their diets.

This book includes chapters relating to new uric acid concepts in tubular transport and the early recognition of renal lesions due to an environmental and genetic predisposition to high blood uric acid. Also covered are the effects of high blood uric acid in preeclampsia, metabolic syndrome, diabetes, high blood pressure in the young, and the relationship between uric acid and vitamin D.

Interesting discussion is included of uric acid as a factor in the acceleration of renal diseases, and the effects of hyperuricemia on the progression of chronic renal failure. The benefits of low uric acid in the prognosis of chronic uremia are also considered. Finally, interesting observations from a study group that achieved low blood uric acid values through specific diets and the correct prescription of old and new drugs are presented.

Recent literature features several papers with substantial information concerning the relationship of acute kidney injury and the rejection of renal transplantation due to hyperuricemia. This latest book in the *Contributions to Nephrology* series offers the reader access to the most up-to-date scientific information, as well as stimulating discussion with which to develop further research in this field. It is hoped that the knowledge provided will help procure new insights into the role of uric acid in renal damage, and how it can be treated and prevented.

Alejandro Treviño-Becerra, Mexico City
Kunitoshi Iseki, Okinawa

Treviño-Becerra A, Iseki K (eds): Uric Acid in Chronic Kidney Disease.
Contrib Nephrol. Basel, Karger, 2018, vol 192, pp 1–7 (DOI: 10.1159/000484271)

Renal Handling of Uric Acid

Jorge Andrade Sierra[a–c] · Milagros M. Flores Fonseca[b]

[a]Department of Physiology, University Health Sciences Center (Centro Universitario de Ciencias de la Salud), University of Guadalajara, Guadalajara, [b]Department of Nephrology and Organ Transplant Unit, Hospital de Especialidades, Centro Medico Nacional de Occidente (CMNO), IMSS, Guadalajara, and [c]Department of Internal Medicine, Civil Hospital of Guadalajara "Dr. Juan I. Menchaca", Guadalajara, México

Abstract

Hyperuricemia occurs in 21.4% of the adult population and is associated with several conditions that increase oxidative stress and contributes to the pathogenesis of inflammatory mechanisms for the development and progression of diseases. Serum blood or urine samples of uric acid levels were used to mainly identify clinical problems, depending on the uric acid pathway alterations, which include synthesis, reabsorption or its excretion. Several proteins that act particularly as transporters (URAT1, GLUT9, 1-NPT1, 1-NPT4, OAT4, 9-MCT9, hUAT1, etc.) have been identified in the recent past involving tubular transport and clearance leading to clinical benefits. Until now, the knowledge of uric acid homeostasis centers its primary investigation on understanding molecular and genetic mechanisms, including the genetic polymorphisms that induce genetic and acquire renal tubular disorder, which increases or diminishes urate excretion.

Introduction

Uric acid is a heterocyclic compound (2,6,8-trihydroxypurine [$C_5H_4N_4O_3$]) and its diprotic acid characteristics include 2 dissociable protons with $pKa_1 \approx 5.4$ and $pKa_2 \approx 10.3$. At physiological human pH, the breakdown of uric acid occurs in 99%, forming acid urate ion in the extracellular fluid, mainly in its circulating form [1, 2].

In a constant neutral blood pH, the index between urate ion and uric acid remains stable and the average concentration of urate levels is close to the solubility limit (6.8 mg/dL). Both terms refer to the total uric acid value (dissociated and undissociated forms) [2]. Even though uric acid excretion happens through the kidneys, the urinary point of neutrality on the pH scale ranges from 4.6 to 8.0 but varies much more in lower urinary pH, increasing in greater proportion its undissociated form because of its poor solubility in aqueous solution [2].

Circulating and Urinary Uric Acid Levels

Humans are adapted to the presence of metabolic waste products, where urate ions are not the exception, and threshold values in men are 1,200 mg/dL, usually higher than that in women. During the fertility timeline, uric acid renal transporters decrease, thereby, producing an imbalance between reabsorption and excretion [3].

Under normal conditions, the kidneys excrete about 70% of total body uric acid production and a smaller proportion is secreted into the intestine and metabolized by gut bacteria in a process termed intestinal uricolysis [1, 2, 4]. In a human urine sample, the reference range of uric acid is typically 620 ± 75.20 mg/dL, which includes the uric acid excretion rate (product of the filtered load) of 0.40 ± 0.09 mg/dL and fractional excretion of urate (FEUA) 7.25 ± 2.98% [1, 2].

FEUA represents the percentage of filtered urate that is excreted in the final urine. It is obtained from urine and plasma samples and calculated as FEUA = $C_{UA}/C_{Cr} \times 100\% = ([U_{UA} \times \text{Urine sample volume}]/P_{UA})/([U_{Cr} \times \text{Urine sample volume}]/P_{Cr}) \times 100\% = (U_{UA} \times P_{Cr})/(P_{UA} \times U_{Cr}) \times 100\%$. Homeostasis between production and excretion of uric acid is determined primarily by urate concentration in blood samples. In normal conditions, reference intervals are between 6.0 and 7.0 mg/dL, primarily gender variations [1]. Increased concentration levels in plasma are known as hyperuricemia and in urine as hyperuricosuria.

Uric Acid Basis

In some mammalian species and other living organisms, uric acid is usually a product of the metabolic breakdown in purine metabolism. Uricase or urate oxidase usually oxidizes to allantoin, a highly hydrolyzed product that is afterwards excreted in urine. Humans have a nonfunctional urate oxidase because of which protein drug formulations do benefit in certain pathological conditions [2].

Humans are not able to oxidize uric acid due to its lack of urate oxidase activity, so the liver is in charge of involving some enzymatic reactions to convert the 2 pu-

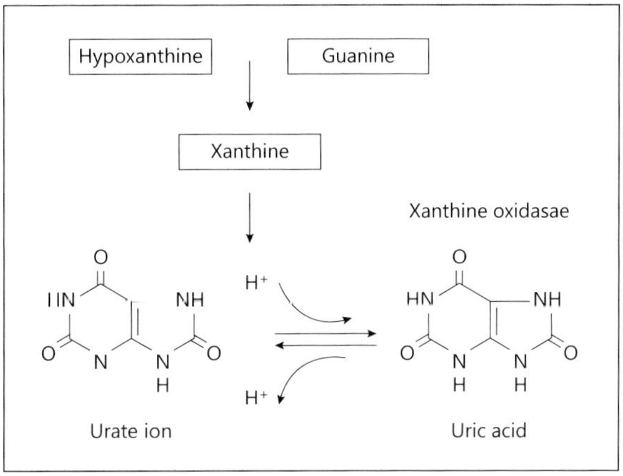

Fig. 1. Oxidation of xanthine by xanthine oxidase to form uric acid.

rine nucleic acids, adenine and guanine, to uric acid. Initially, guanine monophosphate, adenosine monophosphate and inosine monophosphate are converted to nucleosides, inosine and guanosine, and further converted to a purine base, hypoxanthine and guanine, which undergoes chemical processes to form xanthine. Finally, xanthine is oxidized by xanthine oxidase to form uric acid Figure 1.

Tubular Handling and Excretion of Uric Acid

Uric acid has no metabolic response in other tissues; it is known as a metabolic waste product and excreted by the kidneys and the intestine. Urate handling involves kidney and intestine epithelial cells encoded by the ABCG2 gene, an ATP-binding protein, alternatively referred to as Breast Cancer Resistance protein, localized on chromosome 4[5, 6].Two-thirds of the uric acid is expelled by the kidneys, while one-thirds is eliminated by the gastrointestinal tract. Uric acid homeostasis in blood or urine samples is achieved in the form of a complex interplay proposed by Diamond and Paolino [7], which includes glomerular filtration, reabsorptive and secretory transport pathways primarily in the renal proximal tubule cell mediated by incompletely understood molecular mechanisms.

Approximately 99% of uric acid reabsorption occurs in the proximal tubule cell, and 2% left as a percentage filtered to be excreted in the final urine. Reabsorption is primarily accomplished at the S1 segment of the proximal tubule. Following reabsorption, excretion takes place at the S2 segment of the proximal tubule. Post-secretory reabsorption occurs at the S3 segment of the proximal tubule (80% of the excreted urate), and approximately 10% of the filtered uric acid appears to be excreted in the urine [1]. Even though the kidney plays an important role in uric acid balance, bidirectional transport remains partially unknown.

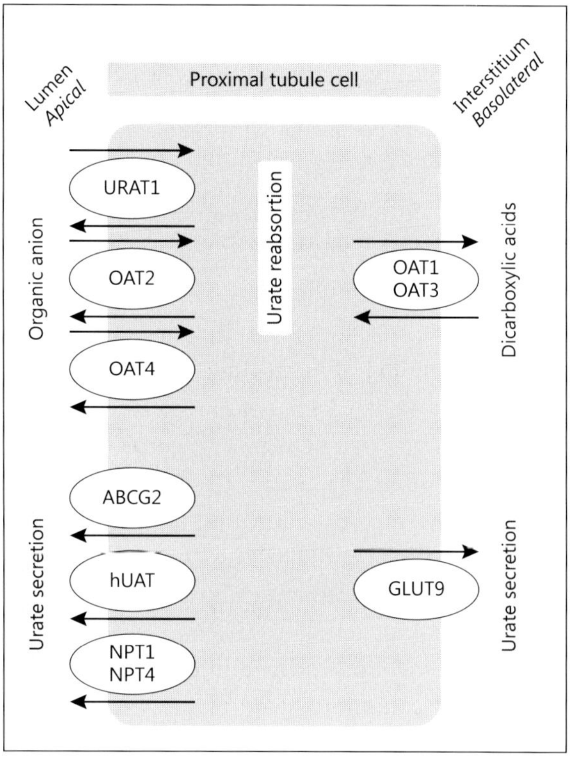

Fig. 2. Transport proteins involved in urate handling in the proximal tubule cell.

Filtered acid uric is reabsorbed by several proteins belonging to the organic anion transporter (OAT) family. The URAT1, a member of the OAT branch, is located on the apical membrane of the renal proximal tubule and encoded by the SLC22A12 gene, which is located on the chromosome 11q13 [2, 8]. URAT1 favours urate ion exchange by anions through the tubule for maintaining electrical balance [9]. Once there is a basolateral entry of urate into the renal proximal tubule cells, it is driven by voltage-dependent urate transport (URAT1v), which is found on the basolateral membrane, encoded by the SLC2A9, and located on chromosome 4 [10, 11]. URAT1v is known as GLUT9, reported initially as a hexose transporter (glucose and fructose) [12]. Two isoforms have been identified: GLUT9L and GLUT9S, localized on the basal and apical membranes, respectively, and they are considered the principal regulators of uric acid in humans [13, 14]. Along the tubule, other molecules favor renal reabsorption of uric acid such as sodium-coupled transporters that codify the gene SLC5A8 [15, 16]. These cotransporters play an independent and sinergical pathway in URAT1 for carboxylic acids including lactate, butyrate, nicotinate, beta-hydroxibutyrate and acetoacetate [17]. Finally, the OAT family, which encodes the SLC22 genes, is localized in the basolateral (OAT 1 and 3) and apical (OAT 2 and 4) membrane of the renal proximal tubules (Fig. 2).

Table 1. Genes and binding transporter on uric acid renal handling

ABCG2 (ATP-binding transporters of purine nucleosides) [6, 23]
SLC17A1 (Sodium-dependent phosphate transporter protein 1-NPT1) [24]
SLC17A3 (Sodium-dependent phosphate transporter protein 1-NPT4) [17]
SLC22A11 (Solute carrier family 22: organic anion/urate transporte-OAT4) [25]
SLC16A9 (Solute Carrier Family 16 Monocarboxylate transporter 9-MCT9) [25]
PDZK1 (URAT1-PDZ-NPT1 domain-containing scaffolding protein) [25, 26]
hUAT1 (Galectine-9 (voltage-sensible urate transport) [27]

Renal handling of uric acid is not just limited to the previous description; conditions associated to hyperuricemia such as gout describe various urate transporters involved in its pathophysiology such as SLC22A12, SLC2A9 [3, 11, 17], and the SLC5A8 [15, 16] as shown in Table 1.

Pathogenic Role of Uric Acid Renal Transport

In the adult population, hyperuricemia occurs in 21.4% [24] and is associated with several conditions that increases oxidative stress (metabolic syndrome, obesity, diabetes, hypertension, renal dysfunction and atherosclerosis); it also contributes to the pathogenesis of inflammatory mechanisms and to the development and progression of co-morbidities (activation of renin – angiotensin system, alteration of intrahepatic fructose metabolism and endothelial dysfunction) [2, 18–20].

Serum blood and urine alterations of uric acid levels mainly identified clinical problems, depending on uric acid synthesis, reabsorption or its excretion. Several proteins that act particularly as transporters (URAT1 and GLUT9) have been identified in recent years involving tubular transport and clearance aimed towards achieving clinical benefits [2]. In addition, these transporters can be affected by some drugs (diuretics, probenecid, losartan, etc.) that act as uricosuric causing alterations on hemodynamic and metabolic processes, which affect uric acid renal excretion [8].

Until now, the knowledge of uric acid homeostasis, centers its primary investigation on understanding molecular and genetic mechanisms, including the genetic polymorphisms that induce genetic and trigger renal tubular disorder, which increases or diminishes urate excretion modifying the function of the transporter proteins (URAT1, GLUT9, 1-NPT1, 1-NPT4, OAT4, 9-MCT9, PDZK1 „URAT1-PDZ-NPT1", hUAT1 or Galectine-9) [3, 11, 17, 21–27].

References

1 Martín NE: Hipouricemia y manejo renal del ácido úrico. Nefrología 2011;31:44–50.

2 Bobulescu IA, Moe OW: Renal transport of uric acid: evolving concepts and uncertainties. Adv Chronic Kidney Dis 2012;19:358–371.

3 Döring A, Gieger C, Mehta D, et al: SLC2A9 influences uric acid concentrations with pronounced sex-specific effects. Nat Genet 2008;40:430–436.

4 Maesaka JK, Fishbane S: Regulation of renal urate excretion: a critical review. Am J Kidney Dis 1998;32:917–933.

5 Ichida K, Matsuo H, Takada T, et al: Decreased extra-renal urate excretion is a common cause of hyperuricemia. Nat Commun 2012;3:764.

6 Huls M, Brown CD, Windass AS, et al: The breast cancer resistance protein transporter ABCG2 is expressed in the human kidney proximal tubule apical membrane. Kidney Int 2008;73:220–225.

7 Diamond HS, Paolino JS: Evidence for a post-secretory reabsorptive site for uric acid in man. J Clin Invest 1973;52:1491–1499.

8 Enomoto A, Kimura H, Chairoungdua A, et al: Molecular identification of a renal urate anion exchanger that regulates blood urate levels. Nature 2002;417:447–452.

9 Koepsell H, Endou H: The SLC22 drug transporter family. Pflugers Arch 2004;447:666–676.

10 Jutabha P, Kanai Y, Hosoyamada M, et al: Identification of a novel voltage-driven organic anion transporter present at apical membrane of renal proximal tubule. J Biol Chem 2003;278:27930–27938.

11 Vitart V, Rudan I, Hayward C, et al: SLC2A9 is a newly identified urate transporter influencing serum urate concentration, urate excretion and gout. Nat Genet 2008;40:437–442.

12 Phay JE, Hussain HB, Moley JF: Cloning and expression analysis of a novel member of the facilitative glucose transporter family, SLC2A9 (GLUT9). Genomics 2000;66:217–220.

13 Augustin R, Carayannopoulos MO, Dowd LO, Phay JE, Moley JF, Moley KH: Identification and characterization of human glucose transporter-like protein-9 (GLUT9): alternative splicing alters trafficking. J Biol Chem 2004;279:16229–16236.

14 Matsuo H, Chiba T, Nagamori S, et al: Mutations in glucose transporter 9 gene SLC2A9 cause renal hypouricemia. Am J Hum Genet 2008;83:744–751.

15 Guggino SE, Aronson PS: Paradoxical effects of pyrazinoate and nicotinate on urate transport in dog renal microvillus membranes. J Clin Invest 1985;76:543–547.

16 Kahn AM: Indirect coupling between sodium and urate transport in the proximal tubule. Kidney Int 1989;36:378–384.

17 Dehghan A, Köttgen A, Yang Q, et al: Association of three genetic loci with uric acid concentration and risk of gout: a genome-wide association study. Lancet 2008;372:1953–1961.

18 Nakagawa T, Tuttle KR, Short RA, Johnson RJ: Hypothesis: fructose-induced hyperuricemia as a causal mechanism for the epidemic of the metabolic syndrome. Nat Clin Pract Nephrol 2005;1:80–86.

19 Choi HK, Curhan G: Soft drinks, fructose consumption, and the risk of gout in men: prospective cohort study. BMJ 2008;336:309–312.

20 Choi JW, Ford ES, Gao X, Choi HK: Sugar-sweetened soft drinks, diet soft drinks, and serum uric acid level: the Third National Health and Nutrition Examination Survey. Arthritis Rheum 2008;59:109–116.

21 Ichida K, Hosoyamada M, Hisatome I, et al: Clinical and molecular analysis of patients with renal hypouricemia in Japan-influence of URAT1 gene on urinary urate excretion. J Am Soc Nephrol 2004;15:164–173.

22 Anzai N, Ichida K, Jutabha P, et al: Plasma urate level is directly regulated by a voltage-driven urate efflux transporter URATv1 (SLC2A9) in humans. J Biol Chem 2008;283:26834–26838.

23 Woodward OM, Köttgen A, Coresh J, Boerwinkle E, Guggino WB, Köttgen M: Identification of a urate transporter, ABCG2, with a common functional polymorphism causing gout. Proc Natl Acad Sci USA 2009;106:10338–10342.

24 Urano W, Taniguchi A, Anzai N, et al: Sodium-dependent phosphate cotransporter type 1 sequence polymorphisms in male patients with gout. Ann Rheum Dis 2010;69:1232–1234.

25 Kolz M, Johnson T, Sanna S, et al: Meta-analysis of 28,141 individuals identifies common variants within five new loci that influence uric acid concentrations. PLoS Genet 2009; 5:e1000504.
26 Endou H, Anzai N: Urate transport across the apical membrane of renal proximal tubules. Nucleosides Nucleotides Nucleic Acids 2008;27:578–584.
27 Lipkowitz MS, Leal-Pinto E, Rappoport JZ, Najfeld V, Abramson RG: Functional reconstitution, membrane targeting, genomic structure, and chromosomal localization of a human urate transporter. J Clin Invest 2001; 107:1103–1115.

Jorge Andrade Sierra, MD, PhD
Department of Physiology, University Health Sciences Center (Centro Universitario de Ciencias de la Salud), University of Guadalajara
Sierra Mojada N°950, Col. Independencia
Guadalajara, Jalisco, CP 44340 (México)
E-Mail jorg_Andrade@hotmail.com

Treviño-Becerra A, Iseki K (eds): Uric Acid in Chronic Kidney Disease.
Contrib Nephrol. Basel, Karger, 2018, vol 192, pp 8–16 (DOI: 10.1159/000484273)

Renal Effects of Hyperuricemia

Carlos Enrique Méndez Landa

Department of Nephrology, General Hospital and Medical Unit Ambulatory Care, Mexican Institute of Social Security, Mexico City, Mexico

Abstract

Background: From a clinical point of view, uric acid has been dismissed as a cause of injury and renal progression, and the mechanisms by which uric acid directly causes renal injury have not been fully understood. Hyperuricemia is associated with metabolic syndrome, diabetes, hypertension, and kidney and cardiovascular diseases. Although it remains controversial whether hyperuricemia is a causal factor for kidney disease, kidneys play a major role in the regulation of serum uric acid levels. ***Summary:*** Similar to the management of other substances, renal uric acid management occurs mainly in the proximal tubule. The elevation of uric acid in blood is mainly due to an increase in its intake or a defect in its secretion. The mechanisms of renal damage go beyond the deposition of crystals at the tubular level; in this sense, renal damage also contributes to the production of chemotactic cytokines, cell proliferation, and inflammation, with the development of afferent arteriolopathy, glomerular hypertrophy and tubulointersticial fibrosis. Nevertheless, whether or not hyperuricemia plays a causal role or simply is a marker arising in the course of each related disorder remains unresolved. Although a strong relationship between hyperuricemia and metabolic syndrome has been established through animal and epidemiological studies, the potential pathophysiological mechanisms by which uric acid contributes to this disease state are just beginning to be explained and clarified. ***Key Messages:*** Experimental studies performed in animals have limitations due to the differences that exist between humans and other mammals in purine metabolism and in renal uric acid handling. Additional experimental studies aimed at evaluating the effects of lowering urate levels on the courses of these disorders are warranted in the future.

Renal Handling of Uric Acid

The renal handling of uric acid involves a complex 4-component system in which uric acid is first filtered and then extensively reabsorbed, followed by tubular secretion and postsecretory reabsorption. Secretion and reabsorption are probably distributed coextensively throughout the proximal and, perhaps, distal tubules, thereby preventing an inordinately high concentration of urate within the tubular lumen at any single location [1].

Most patients with gout have normal excretion rates of uric acid and yet maintain sustained hyperuricemia. This observation implies the presence of an inefficient mechanism for renal tubular excretion of uric acid in these patients. It is known that by using the antituberculous drug pyrazinamide, which is thought to block renal tubular secretion of urate, for a given serum level of uric acid, patients with gout have a lower rate of uric acid secretion than do normal individual. This defect, in essence, requires an increased preload of uric acid in the serum in order that the daily production of uric acid to be excreted by the gouty patient's kidney. So the urate deposit is probably initiated outside the tubular lumen [2].

Experimental Urate Nephropathy

A model for hyperuricemic nephropathy was described by Stavric, Johnson, and Brice. Hyperuricemia and uricosuria were induced in rats fed with uric acid and oxonic acid. After 1 day of hyperuricemia, animals had deposits of uric acid and urate crystals within collecting tubules of the renal papillae, and tubular cells were altered. By 10 days, there was an exudative response with further injury to epithelium [3]. Electron microscopic studies indicate that human neutrophils rapidly ingest monosodium urate crystals. Within neutrophils, the crystals are enclosed phagolvsosomes containing at least one hydrolase, acid phosphatase. There is dissolution of the membrane about the phagolysosome and release of contents into the cytoplasmic matrix leading to the lysis of the neutrophil itself. The urate crystal is thereby free to initiate injury in other cells [4]. Micropuncture studies demonstrate a decrease in the single-nephron glomerular filtration rate (GFR) associated with a twofold increase in tubular hydrostatic pressure. Pathologic examination shows numerous white streaks throughout the medulla and pyramids caused by intratubular deposition of acid uric and urate crystals. Secondary tubular atrophy, infiltration of inflammatory cells, and interstitial fibrosis have also been reported [2, 4].

Johnson's work group has found that raising the uric acid level could induce oxidative stress and endothelial dysfunction, resulting in the development of both systemic and glomerular hypertension in association with elevated renal vascular resistance and reduced renal blood flow. In normal rats, there was activation of the renin-angiotensin system, with the development of vascular disease of the afferent arteriolar system (arteriolosclerosis) and glomerular hypertrophy, and over time mild interstitial disease and glomerulosclerosis [5].

There are 2 different types of renal diseases induced by uric acid: acute uric acid nephropathy and chronic urate nephropathy.

Acute Uric Acid Nephropathy

Although it is widely recognized that markedly elevated levels of uric acid can cause acute renal failure (ARF), by crystal deposits, the possibility that uric acid may affect renal outcomes at concentrations that do not lead to tubular obstruction have not been considered.

Tumor lysis syndrome (TLS) is a major metabolic disorder, which is frequently found after cell destruction produced in most cases subsequent to the initiation of cytotoxic therapy, used in a variety of cancers including lymphoma and leukemia, which could lead to acute uric acid nephropathy [6]. Rapid cell destruction causes an abrupt release of intracellular ions, nucleic acids, proteins, and their metabolites into the extracellular space. Hyperuricemia is the key factor in the pathogenesis of TLS. The lysis results in the release of large amounts of nucleic acids, which are quantitatively converted to uric acid and must be excreted by the kidney. Crystallization damage occurs in TLS when calcium phosphate, uric acid, and xanthine precipitate in the renal tubules and result in inflammation and obstruction. Uric acid can induce renal damage not only by intrarenal crystallization but also by independent crystallization mechanisms such as vasoconstriction, the inability to self-regulate, decreases in renal blood flow, production of oxidation, and inflammation. Initially uricosuria is present, often manifested by uric acid crystals in the urinary sediment. Microscopic or gross hematuria is seen occasionally. It is common for it to present as an acute oliguric renal injury. The pathologic findings in the kidney result from the deposition of uric acid crystals in the collecting ducts, renal pelvis, and ureters, which produce hydronephrosis [1, 7].

There are several mechanisms by which uric acid may contribute to ARF. First, renal vasoconstriction by inhibition of nitric oxide synthase, reduction in endothelial cell nitric oxide, and stimulation of the renin-angiotensin system lead to ARF. Second, antiangiogenic properties (inhibition of endothelial cell proliferation and migration, stimulation of endothelial cell apoptosis) result in ARF. Third, proinflammatory properties (stimulation of monocyte chemoattractant protein-1 and C-reactive protein, activation of nuclear factor-kappa B and p38 mitogen-activated protein kinase) and pro-oxidative properties (stimulation of oxidants and peroxynitrite-associated radicals), and last alteration of renal autoregulation all lead to ARF [8].

On the other hand, diuretics have been used commonly in the management of ARF to aid in the management of extracellular volume. Diuretics stimulate the reabsorption of uric acid in the proximal tubule, both by inducing direct effects of diuretics on the renal transporters and by causing a reduction in renal perfusion, which secondarily stimulates proximal sodium and urate reabsorption [9].

Hyperuricemia and Chronic Kidney Disease

Chronic urate nephropathy was primarily seen in the past in patients with tophaceous gout. However, it is currently thought to be uncommon and some feel that the diagnosis cannot be made on clinical grounds in the absence of renal biopsy [10]. Most studies documented that an elevated serum uric acid level independently predicts the development of chronic kidney disease (CKD). The specific mechanism(s) by which uric acid may be causing these effects has been studied. One of the more striking findings is that uric acid is a prooxidant inside the cell where it can induce stimulation of NADPH oxidases with the induction of mitochondrial dysfunction. Uric acid can also induce endothelial dysfunction via a variety of mechanisms. In addition to the effect already commented on vascular smooth muscle cells with the production of chemotactic and oxidizing factors and the activation of RAS [11].

The role of uric acid in the development and progression of CKD has been evaluated by several epidemiological studies. There is evidence that elevated uric acid concentration may be a predictor of progression, especially in diabetes and IgA nephropathy [12].

In diabetes, serum uric acid is often low because of the effects of glycosuria in increasing urate excretion. As a result, it is possible to find a low serum uric acid level in subjects with uncontrolled glucose. In subjects with type 1 diabetes, an elevated serum uric acid level, even when within the normal range, is a strong predictor for the development of both incipient (microalbuminuric) and established (albuminuric) diabetic nephropathy. It also predicts the development of CKD, the development and progression of CKD in subjects with type 2 diabetes [13, 14].

In chronic urate nephropathy the deposition of sodium urate crystals in the medullary interstitium is appreciated. This results in a chronic inflammatory response, similar to that seen with microtophus formation elsewhere in the body, potentially leading to interstitial fibrosis and CKD. Although urate crystals in the renal medulla are demonstrable on biopsy, the clinical features of chronic urate nephropathy are nonspecific: renal functional impairment, bland urinary sediment, mild proteinuria, and serum urate concentrations are often higher than expected in terms of the degree of impaired renal function. Nevertheless, it is difficult to separate hyperuricemia from the other causes of renal impairment that can occur in patients with hyperuricemia, such as hypertension and diabetes mellitus [15].

Hyperuricemia and Hypertension, Implications in Renal Damage
The association between hyperuricemia and hypertension is accepted and supported by the following observations:

- Hyperuricemia prevalence of approximately 20–40% in untreated hypertensive patients and 50–70% in hypertensive patients treated or with renal impairment.
- Gout prevalence of 2–12% in hypertensive patients.
- Prevalence of hypertension of 25–50% in patients with gout.
- Increasing prevalence of hyperuricemia with increasing blood pressure in the general population.
- Increasing risk for development of hypertension with increasing baseline serum urate levels [16].

Despite these assertions, the conflicting results of different studies avoid establishing a cause effect. Grahame and Scott [17] documented that the high prevalence of hypertension in patients with gout had a strong association with obesity more than with the duration of gout. In the Ischemic Heart Disease Study of Israel, it was documented that only 1% of the variation in blood pressure could be explained by serum urate [18]. In other studies, the association of elevated serum levels of uric acid with the future development of hypertension has been documented [19, 20].

From animal models, Feig [21] has suggested a 2-phase mechanism through which hyperuricemia leads to the development of hypertension. Initially, uric acid induces vasoconstriction by the activation of the renin-angiotensin system and reduction of circulating nitric oxide, which can be reversed by lowering uric acid. In the second phase, uric acid mediated arteriolosclerosis. Uric acid uptake into vascular smooth muscle cells causes the activation and elaboration of production of growth factor and monocyte chemoattractant protein-1. It causes cellular proliferation and secondary arteriolosclerosis that impair pressure natriuresis, causing sodium-sensitive hypertension [22]. This observation has been previously described, finding that uric acid stimulates the proliferation of vascular smooth muscle cells, precisely because of the expression of this cytokine. Among the alterations in the renal structure that have been described are glomerular hypertrophy, glomerular hypertension, afferent arteriolar sclerosis, tubulointerstitial injury along with monocyte infiltration, and the development of mild vascular disease involving the preglomerular arterioles [23, 24].

Hyperuricemia and Metabolic Syndrome

It is well accepted that individuals who are hyperuricemic and hyperlipidemic, particularly those with abdominal obesity, may be a high-risk group for cardiovascular events: reviewed evidence supports inclusion of hyperuricemia resulting from impaired renal uric acid clearance as an intrinsic component of the metabolic syndrome of hyperinsulinemia and resistance to insulin action.

Several epidemiological investigations have confirmed the association of hyperuricemia with metabolic syndrome. Some have suggested that uric acid may simply be a consequence of the increased uric acid absorption in the proximal tubule secondary to hyperinsulinemia, and others believe that uric acid may predict the development of metabolic syndrome, obesity, and diabetes [25].

A fructose-rich diet can raise uric acid production and induce the components of metabolic syndrome through mechanisms independent of energy intake or weight gain. These effects are not observed with a glucose-rich diet. Recently, uric acid also was found to have a causal role in the metabolic syndrome that was induced experimentally by fructose. Fructose rapidly raises uric acid as a consequence of activation of fructokinase with ATP consumption, intracellular phosphate depletion, and stimulation of AMP deaminase. Lowering uric acid in fructose-fed rats ameliorates much of the metabolic syndrome, including a reduction in blood pressure, serum triglycerides, hyperinsulinemia, and weight gain. The rise in uric acid after fructose ingestion likely has a significant role in inducing insulin resistance via its effect to lower nitric oxide and also possibly by a direct effect of uric acid on the adipocytes [26].

Data also support an association between hyperuricemia and endothelial dysfunction in human and importantly, support the fact that this endothelial dysfunction can be reversed by the administration of allopurinol in animal model as well as in human subjects. Since oxidative stress in adipocytes has been considered a major factor of insulin resistance, hyperuricemia-induced oxidative stress in adipose tissue might play a key role in these dysregulations [27].

Hyperuricemia and Renal Transplant

It has already been commented that uric acid is involved in endothelial dysfunction, proliferation of vascular smooth muscle, and stimulation of profibrotic and inflammatory cytokines. The evidence addressing the association between elevated uric acid with GFR decline in renal transplant recipients in whom hyperuricemia is highly prevalent is contradictory. While some studies did not document an association between the level of uric acid and the decline of GFR in KTR, there are others that report the association to range from a slight to a strong one. Cyclosporine is also known to raise the uric acid level, and we found that the renal disease induced by cyclosporine could be worsened by raising the uric acid level and lessened by lowering it [28].

In a review, Bellomo [29] summarized epidemiological and interventional studies that demonstrated the association between elevated uric acid level and its consequences on renal graft function. Concluding that randomized controlled trials of urate lowering therapy are badly needed in this population of patients, to establish whether preservation of renal function and prolongation of graft survival can be achieved.

Hart and et al. [30], identified the association between uric acid and the primary composite outcome of doubling of interstitium or ESRD from interstitial fibrosis and tubular atrophy, and also found that a 1 mg/dL increase in time-varying uric acid was associated with a 2.39 mL/min lower final GFR but not with the secondary outcome of creatinine doubling, ESRD, or death.

Conclusions

Most studies have suggested that uric acid may also play a role in in the progression of hypertension, cardiovascular disease, metabolic syndrome, and renal disease. Animal studies demonstrate that elevated uric acid level causes hypertension and endothelial dysfunction, arteriolopathy, and CKD and studies in human suggest an association of hyperuricemia with CKD, hypertension, and cardiovascular disease. It is clear that uric acid is an important participant in the development of kidney damage. In the general population, an elevation of uric acid is correlated with decreased renal function. Uric acid is also associated with renal dysfunction in hypertensive patients, as well as with microalbuminuria in type 2 diabetes. Although they are better understood, the mechanisms by which the uric acid is cause of kidney damage.

References

1 Beck LH: Requiem for gouty nephropathy. Kidney Int 1986;30:280–287.
2 Waisman J, Mwasi LM, Bluestone R, Klinenberg JR: Acute hyperuricemic nephropathy in rats. An electron microscopic study. Am J Pathol 1975;81:367–378.
3 Hoffstein S, Weissmann G: Mechanisms of lysosomal enzyme release from leukocytes. IV. Interaction of monosodium urate crystals with dogfish and human leukocytes. Arthritis Rheum 1973;18:153–165.
4 Fogo AB, Kashgarian M: Tubulointerstitial Diseases, Urate Nephropathy, in Diagnostic Atlas of Renal Pathology, ed 3. Philadelphia, Elseiver, 2017, p 446.
5 Johnson R, Nakagawa T, Jalal D, Sanchez-Lozada LG, Kang DH, Ritz E: Uric acid and chronic kidney disease: which is chasing which? Nephrol Dial Transplant 2013;28: 2221–2228.
6 González-Sanchez AG, Rubio-Jurado B, et al: Síndrome de lisis tumoral. El Residente 2013; 8:35–43.
7 Scott CH, Jones DP, Ching-Hon P: The tumor lisys syndrome. N Engl J Med 2011:364: 1844–1854.
8 Ejaz AA, Mu W, Kang DH, Roncal C, Sautin YY, Henderson G, Tabah-Fisch I, Keller B, Beaver TM, Nakagawa T, Johnson RJ: Could uric acid have a role in acute renal failure? Clin J Am Soc Nephrol 2007;2:16–21.
9 Steele TH, Oppenheimer S: Factors affecting urate excretion following diuretic administration in man. Am J Med 1969;47:564–574.
10 Moe OW: Posing the question again: does chronic uric acid nephropathy exist? J Am Soc Nephrol 2010;21:395–397.
11 Sánchez-Lozada LG, Lanaspa MA, Cristóbal-García M, García-Arroyo F, Soto V, Cruz-Robles D, Nakagawa T, Yu MA, Kang DH, Johnson RJ: Uric acid-induced endothelial dysfunction is associated with mitochondrial alterations and decreased intracellular ATP concentrations. Nephron Exp Nephrol 2012; 121:e71–e77.
12 Treviño-Becerra A: Hypertriglyceridaemia and hyperuricaemia in IgA nephropathy. Nephrol Dial Transplant 2011;16:639.
13 Ficociello LH, Rosolowsky ET, Niewczas MA, Maselli NJ, Weinberg JM, Aschengrau A, Eckfeldt JH, Stanton RC, Galecki AT, Doria A, Warram JH, Krolewski AS: High-normal serum uric acid increases risk of early progressive renal function loss in type 1 diabetes: results of a 6-year follow-up. Diabetes Care 2010;33:1337–1343.
14 Johnson RJ, Kivlighn SD, Kim YG, et al: Reappraisal of the pathogenesis and consequences of hyperuricemia in hypertension, cardiovascular disease, and renal disease. Am J Kidney Dis 1999;33:225–234.
15 Jossa F, Farinaro E, Panico S, Krogh V, Celentano E, Galasso R, Mancini M, Trevisan M: Serum uric acid and hypertension: the Olivetti heart study. J Hum Hypertens 1994; 8:677–681.
16 Kahn HA, Medalie JH, Neufeld HN, Riss E, Goldbourt U: The incidence of hypertension and associated factors: the Israel ischemic heart disease study. Am Heart J 1972;84:171–182.
17 Grahame R, Scott JT: Clinical survey of 354 patients with gout. Ann Rheum Dis 1970;29: 461–468.
18 Nakanishi N, Okamoto M, Yoshida H, Matsuo Y, Suzuki K, Tatara K: Serum uric acid and risk for development of hypertension and impaired fasting glucose or type II diabetes in Japanese male office workers. Eur J Epidemiol 2003;18:523–530.
19 Hunt SC, Stephenson SH, Hopkins PN, Williams RR: Predictors of an increased risk of future hypertension in Utah. A screening analysis. Hypertension 1991;17(6 pt 2):969–976.
20 Kanellis J, Watanabe S, Li JH, Kang DH, Li P, Nakagawa T, Wamsley A, Sheikh-Hamad D, Lan HY, Feng L, Johnson RJ: Uric acid stimulates monocyte chemoattractant protein-1 production in vascular smooth muscle cells via mitogen-activated protein kinase and cyclooxygenase-2. Hypertension 2003;41:1287–1293.
21 Feig DI: The role of uric acid in the pathogenesis of hypertension in the young. J Clin Hypertension 2012;14:346–352.

22 Mazzali M, Kanellis J, Han L, Feng L, Xia YY, Chen Q, Kang DH, Gordon KL, Watanabe S, Nakagawa T, Lan HY, Johnson RJ: Hyperuricemia induces a primary renal arteriolopathy in rats by a blood pressure-independent mechanism. Am J Physiol Renal Physiol 2002;282:F991–F997.
23 Nakagawa T, Mazzali M, Kang DH, Sánchez-Lozada LG, Herrera-Acosta J, Johnson RJ: Uric acid – a uremic toxin? Blood Purif 2006; 24:67–70.
24 Soltani Z, Rasheed K, Kapusta DR, Reisin E: Potential role of uric acid in metabolic syndrome, hypertension, kidney injury, and cardiovascular diseases: is it time for reappraisal? Curr Hypertens Rep 2013;15:175–181.
25 Nakagawa T, Hu H, Zharikov S, Tuttle KR, Short RA, Glushakova O, Ouyang X, Feig DI, Block ER, Herrera-Acosta J, Patel JM, Johnson RJ: A causal role for uric acid in fructose-induced metabolic syndrome. Am J Physiol Renal Physiol 200;290:F625–F631.
26 Khosla UM, et al: Hyperuricemia induces endothelial dysfunction. Kidney Int 2005;67: 1739–1742.
27 Akgul A: Is uric acid a predictive factor for graft dysfunction in renal transplant recipients? Transplant Proc 2007;39:1023–1026.
28 Haririan A, et al: Association of serum uric acid with graft survival after kidney transplantation: a time-varying analysis. Am J Transplant 2011;11:1943–1950.
29 Bellomo G: Asymptomatic hyperuricemia following renal transplantation. World J Nephrol 2015;4:324–329.
30 Hart A, Jackson S, Kasiske BL, Mauer MS, Najafian B, Matas AJ, Spong R, Ibrahim HN: Uric acid and allograft loss from interstitial fibrosis/tubular atrophy: post hoc analysis from the angiotensin II blockade in chronic allograft nephropathy trial. Transplantation 2014;97:1066–1071.

Carlos Enrique Méndez Landa
Department of Nephrology, General Hospital and Medical Unit Ambulatory Care
Elpidio Cortes Street, San Pedro Xalpa Colony, Azcapotzalco
02719, Mexico City (Mexico)
E-Mail ashkeloningvar@gmail.com

Treviño-Becerra A, Iseki K (eds): Uric Acid in Chronic Kidney Disease.
Contrib Nephrol. Basel, Karger, 2018, vol 192, pp 17–24 (DOI: 10.1159/000484274)

The Pathophysiology of Uric Acid on Renal Diseases

L. Gabriela Sánchez-Lozada

Laboratory of Renal Physiopathology, Department of Nephrology, Instituto Nacional de Cardiología Ignacio Chávez, Mexico City, Mexico

Abstract

Background: Asymptomatic hyperuricemia was regarded as a marker and considered secondary to some pathological conditions such as hypertension. During the last 16 years, a vast amount of experimental work has shown that uric acid can cause intracellular alterations that lead to cardiovascular, renal, and metabolic disease. Epidemiological and clinical studies support this notion in specific populations. However, the clinical studies done so far are of such a small number that it is difficult to reach a consensus in regard to the benefit of treating asymptomatic hyperuricemia. ***Summary:*** Mild hyperuricemia in rodents induces hypertension associated to renal microvascular disease, tubulointerstitial inflammation, vasoconstriction, and glomerular hypertension. The cellular mechanisms that lead to those outcomes require an increase in intracellular concentrations of uric acid inducing oxidative stress that then activates the synthesis and secretion of proinflammatory factors and vasoconstrictive substances, and diminishes the bioavailability of nitric oxide produced by eNOS. Uric acid also induces proliferation, senescence, and fat accumulation or inhibits insulin secretion, depending on the cell type. Extracellular uric acid can act as an antioxidant; however, when it crystallizes it also induces the activation of prooxidant and proinflammatory pathways resulting in renal lesion. ***Key Messages:*** Experimental evidence shows that uric acid is a true mediator for cardiovascular, renal, and metabolic diseases. However, there is still need for greater and well-controlled intervention studies in humans to define whether treating asymptomatic hyperuricemia is worthwhile or not.

Introduction

The first associations between hyperuricemia and cardiovascular and renal disease date to the 19th century. The first findings were described in gouty patients in whom "interstitial nephritis in almost the whole parenchyma that resulted in the destruction of glomeruli, tubules, and arterioles" was found [1]. It was thought that uric acid also attacked the arteries of other tissues and caused hypertension [1]. In the 20th century, the term gouty nephropathy was coined to describe the renal lesions observed in a vast proportion of patients with gout. Nevertheless, the notion of "gouty nephropathy" was abandoned, as the focal crystal deposition of uric acid seen in gout could not account for the diffuse nature of the kidney lesions characterized by microvascular disease, interstitial fibrosis, and glomerulosclerosis. Moreover, such lesions are also associated with aging and long-term hypertension. Thus, it was thought that the chronic renal damage observed in gouty patients was related to those factors. In the course of years, several epidemiological studies consistently found that hyperuricemia strongly associated with chronic renal tubulointerstitial disease and cardiovascular disease, and that it even had a predictive value for hypertension and coronary disease. Also, studies in patients with familial juvenile hyperuricemic nephropathy showed that decreased excretion of uric acid and hyperuricemia preceded the onset of renal disease and early treatment with allopurinol retarded renal damage [2–4]. As hyperuricemia mostly results from decreased fractional excretion of uric acid, it was suggested that if uric acid were toxic per se, the site of first involvement would be the kidney, and therefore it would be valuable to test this hypothesis with an experimental model.

A Model for Mild Hyperuricemia

As renal and cardiovascular involvement associated with hyperuricemia was detected after long-term exposure to increased concentrations of serum uric acid, it was hard to establish whether hyperuricemia was a marker of disease or a true causal factor in humans; therefore, a model of primary hyperuricemia was needed. The first challenge to solve was the fact that metabolism of uric acid differs between man and rodents; this is because in the former, UA is the last product of purine degradation pathway, while the latter expresses an uricase in the liver, which further degrades UA to 5-hydroxyisourate and then allantoin. A knockout mouse for uricase was developed, but the inactivation of this enzyme was lethal, as mice died at a young age due to obstructive acute renal failure caused

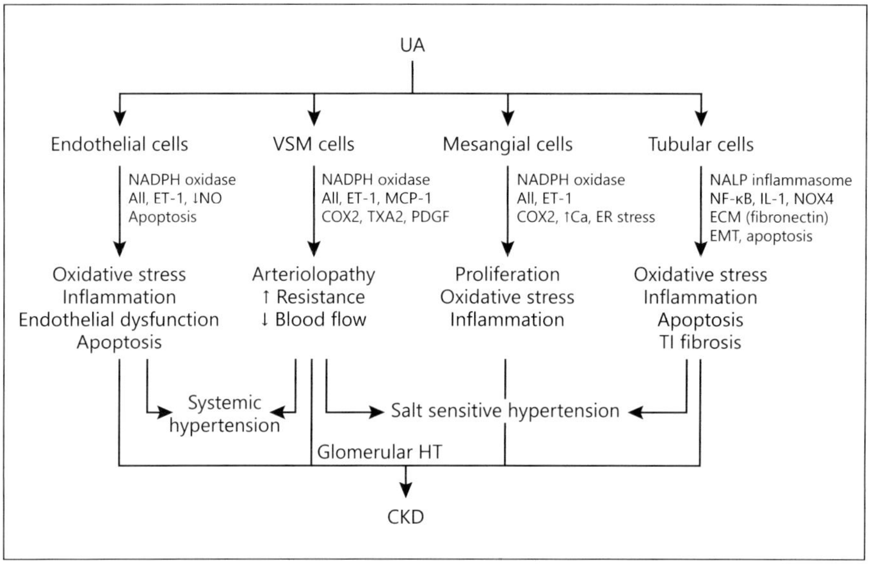

Fig. 1. Proposed mechanisms by which uric acid (UA) causes Ht and CKD. Increased intracellular concentrations of UA affect endothelial, vascular smooth muscle (VSMC), mesangial, and tubular cells by inducing a prooxidant environment that activates proinflammatory, proliferative, senescence, and profibrotic pathways as well as endothelial dysfunction and the synthesis and secretion of vasoconstrictors. The activation of all these damaging pathways leads to systemic hypertension, which with time becomes salt-sensitive, and CKD.

by UA precipitation in renal tubules [5]. Therefore, this model did not reflect the progressive nature of long-term hyperuricemia (HU). A better model was developed by the blockade of uricase with oxonic acid [6]. Administration of this inhibitor on diet induced a rise in serum UA of 1.5–2 times that not precipitated in renal tubules. Hyperuricemic rats developed hypertension after 3 weeks, and this effect was prevented or improved by the concomitant administration of allopurinol or benziodarone to prevent UA synthesis or increase its urine excretion, respectively, or by oxonic acid withdrawal [6]. Also, hyperuricemia induced renal injury. Thus, markers of inflammation (ED-1+ cells and osteopontin) and fibrosis (collagen type III) were significantly increased in tubulointerstitium. Moreover, HU activated the renal renin-angiotensin system and inhibited NOS1 expression. Those findings were suggestive of renal vasoconstriction. Thus, enalapril and arginine administration prevented hypertension as well as the renal disease in HU rats [6]. Later on, it was shown that HU induced afferent arteriolopathy, characterized by the thickening of the media and an increased arteriolar area, which was independent of systemic hypertension but dependent on the activation of the intrarenal renin-angiotensin system

[7]. Preglomerular vascular disease, ischemia, renal inflammation, and tubulointerstitial disease are conditions that result in salt-sensitive hypertension. In agreement, it was shown that the arteriolopathy and the tubulointerstitial changes secondary to HU, induced in the long-term salt-sensitivity was independent of serum uric acid concentrations [8].

Also, it was found that oxonic acid-induced HU resulted in higher blood pressure and greater renal damage in 5 out of 6 remnant kidney rats characterized by greater fibrosis, inflammation, and microvascular damage. Co-treatment with allopurinol blocked those alterations [9]. Therefore, long-term HU causes Chronic kidney disease (CKD) and also accelerates established CKD. Other models in which the pathogenic role of HU has been disclosed are cyclosporine-induced renal injury [10], diabetic nephropathy [11], and acute kidney injury [12, 13].

Renal Hemodynamics in Hyperuricemia

Microvascular renal lesions are associated with the progression of renal damage by altering the autoregulatory response to blood pressure and/or by reducing the blood flow inducing ischemia [14]. Thus, the finding that HU caused afferent arteriolopathy led to the study on whether this lesion had functional implications. By using renal micropuncture techniques, it was found that oxonic acid-induced HU resulted in renal vasoconstriction with a significant increase in afferent and efferent resistances and reduction in single nephron plasma flow, single nephron glomerular filtration rate, and ultrafiltration coefficient (Kf) [15, 16]. An additional consequence of afferent arteriolopathy was the loss of autoregulatory capacity as was disclosed by the transmission of systemic hypertension to glomerular capillaries resulting in glomerular hypertension. Concomitant treatment with allopurinol to OA-treated rats prevented arteriolopathy and the alterations of renal hemodynamics. Moreover, significant positive correlations were found between the afferent arteriole wall area and serum uric acid, and glomerular pressure [15, 16]. It was also concluded that the blockade of the deleterious pathways induced by HU, such as the treatments with antioxidant or l-arginine, provided benefit, and therefore prevented the structural and renal hemodynamic changes induced by HU.

Renal hemodynamic alterations were also studied in 5/6 nephrectomy HU rats [16]. This model is characterized by systemic hypertension and increased renal blood perfusion and hyperfiltration due to a significant increase in glomerular pressure that results from the loss of the autoregulatory capacity in the afferent arteriole [14]. In this setting, HU produced profound renal vasoconstriction with a fall of 40% in single nephron glomerular filtration rate and Kf. There was also a higher proportional increase in afferent resistance than efferent resistance. Despite the intense preglomerular vasoconstriction, glomerular hypertension remained high, and renal damage was accelerated. Therefore, 5/6 nephrectomy rats had higher blood pressure, greater proteinuria, and inflammatory infiltration in comparison to the non-hyperuricemic group. Also, the concomitant treatment with allopurinol prevented the additional renal damage induced by HU in 5/6 nephrectomy rats [16].

In humans, it has been reported that HU is associated with renal microvascular damage, increased renal resistive index, afferent vasoconstriction in healthy subjects, CKD and hypertensive patients [17–19]. HU is also an independent predictor for the development of AKI in several clinical settings.

Damaging Intracellular Pathways Induced by Uric Acid

The common association between uric acid and tissue damage is by means of its extracellular precipitation, similar to what occurs in joints in gout. However, the studies conducted involving mild hyperuricemic animals showed that the rise in intracellular concentrations of UA initiates a cascade of pathways that lead to hypertension, kidney damage, and metabolic alterations.

Soluble UA enters into cells through transporters including URAT1 and organic anion transporters such as OAT 1, 2, 3, 4, and 10. Inhibition of UA transport with probenecid or benziodarone is capable of blocking its toxic effects in vitro, in vivo, as well as in clinical studies [20, 21]. In addition, in several cell types, there is evidence of bidirectional transport of UA [20]. Interestingly, the expression and function (intake or secretion) of the different UA transporters were found to vary according to the organ and species [22], and there is also evidence of interaction among the various UA transporters to regulate systemic UA concentrations [23]. On the other hand, intracellular concentrations of UA may also increase by stimulating its synthesis by xanthine oxidase. Some enzymatic defects resulting from genetic mutations, such as in Lesch-Nyman syndrome, result in UA overproduction. However, environmental factors play a major role; thus, diets rich in fructose or purines, as well as lead exposure can contribute to increasing the synthesis of UA.

Once UA intracellular concentrations increase, via cellular uptake or increased synthesis, the studies suggest that the first step in the deleterious path is the increase in oxidative stress by stimulating NADPH oxidase activity. This primary effect seems to be preserved among several cell types as it has been found in vascular smooth muscle cells, endothelial cells, adipocytes, pancreatic cells, hepatocytes, cardiac fibroblasts, renal tubule, and mesangial cells [24–28]. The increase in intracellular oxidative stress stimulates protein kinases (MAPK's, ERK 1/2), proinflammatory transcription factors (NF-kB), and proliferative factors (PDGF, TGF-b) [24–28]. Stimulation of such pathways then induces the synthesis of vasoconstrictors (Angiotensin II, endothelin-1, thromboxane), proinflammatory factors (MCP-1, PCR), and NLRP3 inflammasome activation with IL-1β secretion. In addition, mitochondrial and endoplasmic reticulum alterations have been described in several cell types [24–28]. UA also induces endothelial dysfunction by reducing NO bioavailability and endothelial cells senescence and apoptosis. In summary, UA activation of damaging pathways has different outcomes that depend on the cell type; thus, in renal tubular and mesangial cells, inflammation and dysfunction are induced, in VSMC, inflammation and proliferation are induced, in endothelial cells, dysfunction and senescence are induced, in hepatocytes, the oxidation of fatty acids is blocked and fatty acid synthesis is promoted, in adipocytes, adiponectin synthesis is inhibited, in pancreatic cells, insulin production is inhibited, and in cardiac fibroblasts, the synthesis of profibrotic molecules is induced [24–28].

On the other hand, extracellular UA can also induce damage. UA solubility is low in physiological fluids, ~6.8–7.0 mg/dL. Individuals with higher concentrations of UA have a supersaturated plasma uric acid concentration, and this condition predisposes to the formation of monosodium urate crystals, although others factors also participate in the initiation of crystallization, since not all hyperuricemic patients develop gout [29]. In the kidney, increased fractional excretion of UA in association with an acidic urine leads to the formation of UA crystals, such as is the case of tumor lysis syndrome, and more recently, this mechanism has also been described as a potential causal factor for the nephropathy from nontraditional causes in Central America, named Mesoamerican Nephropathy [30]. Uric acid crystal-mediated damage includes the activation of tissue macrophages with increased secretion of IL-1β and neutrophil influx [29]. Upon infiltration, neutrophils are further activated by the crystals, producing additional inflammatory mediators [29]. When phagocytized, urate crystals activate the NLRP3 inflammasome, which induces maturation and secretion of IL-1β, and a downstream cascade of inflammation mediated by cytokines, prostanoids, and other molecules [31]. This process would be associated with a couple of kidney diseases, including Mesoamerican Nephropathy and IgA nephropathy. In these diseases, hyperuricemia and uricosuria were found to be related to interstitial fibrosis and tubular atrophy respectively [30, 32–34].

Interestingly, extracellular UA can also function as an antioxidant and exerts neuroprotective effects in acute brain ischemia as well as in other CNS diseases [35]. Thus, regional cellular phenotypes can respond differently to UA.

Conclusions

Experimental studies have shown that uric acid is not an inert waste product of purines catabolism as was previously thought. Instead, it is a pleiotropic molecule with the capacity of inducing deleterious intracellular pathways that result in hypertension, renal lesion, cardiovascular alterations, and metabolic disturbances. In addition, extracellular uric acid can function as an antioxidant, when precipitates also stimulate prooxidant and proinflammatory pathways. However, there are no clinical studies so far that support the use of uric acid-lowering therapy to treat asymptomatic hyperuricemia.

References

1 Davis NS: The cardio-vascular and renal relations and manifestations of gout. JAMA 1897;XXIX:261–262.
2 McBride MB, et al: Presymptomatic detection of familial juvenile hyperuricaemic nephropathy in children. Pediatr Nephrol 1998;12:357–364.
3 McBride MB, et al: Efficacy of allopurinol in ameliorating the progressive renal disease in familial juvenile hyperuricaemic nephropathy (FJHN). A six-year update. Adv Exp Med Biol 1998;431:7–11.
4 Fairbanks LD, et al: Early treatment with allopurinol in familial juvenile hyerpuricaemic nephropathy (FJHN) ameliorates the long-term progression of renal disease. QJM 2002;95:597–607.
5 Wu X, et al: Hyperuricemia and urate nephropathy in urate oxidase-deficient mice. Proc Natl Acad Sci 1994;91:742–746.
6 Mazzali M, et al: Elevated uric acid increases blood pressure in the rat by a novel crystal-independent mechanism. Hypertension 2001;38:1101–1106.
7 Mazzali M, et al: Hyperuricemia induces a primary renal arteriolopathy in rats by a blood pressure-independent mechanism. Am J Physiol Renal Physiol 2002;282:F991–F997.
8 Watanabe S, et al: Uric acid, hominoid evolution, and the pathogenesis of salt-sensitivity. Hypertension 2002;40:355–360.
9 Kang DH, et al: A role for uric acid in the progression of renal disease. J Am Soc Nephrol 2002;13:2888–2897.
10 Mazzali M, et al: Hyperuricemia exacerbates chronic cyclosporine nephropathy. Transplantation 2001;71:900–905.
11 Komers R, et al: Effects of xanthine oxidase inhibition with febuxostat on the development of nephropathy in experimental type 2 diabetes. Br J Pharmacol 2016;173:2573–2588.
12 Omori H, et al: Use of xanthine oxidase inhibitor febuxostat inhibits renal interstitial inflammation and fibrosis in unilateral ureteral obstructive nephropathy. Clin Exp Nephrol 2012;16:549–556.
13 Tsuda H, et al: Febuxostat suppressed renal ischemia-reperfusion injury via reduced oxidative stress. Biochem Biophys Res Commun 2012;427:266–272.
14 Sanchez-Lozada LG, et al: Glomerular hemodynamic changes associated with arteriolar lesions and tubulointerstitial inflammation. Kidney Int Suppl 2003;86:S9–S14.
15 Sanchez-Lozada LG, et al: Mild hyperuricemia induces glomerular hypertension in normal rats. Am J Physiol Renal Physiol 2002;283:F1105–F1110.
16 Sanchez-Lozada LG, et al: Mild hyperuricemia induces vasoconstriction and maintains glomerular hypertension in normal and remnant kidney rats. Kidney Int 2005;67:237–247.
17 Kohagura K, et al: An association between uric acid levels and renal arteriolopathy in chronic kidney disease: a biopsy-based study. Hypertens Res 2013;36:43–49.

18 Uedono H, et al: Relationship between serum uric acid levels and intrarenal hemodynamic parameters. Kidney Blood Press Res 2015;40: 315–322.
19 Geraci G, et al: Association between uric acid and renal hemodynamics: pathophysiological implications for renal damage in hypertensive patients. J Clin Hyperten 2016;18:1007–1014.
20 Mandal A, Mount DB: The molecular physiology of uric acid homeostasis. Ann Rev Physiol 2015;77:1–23.
21 Johnson RJ, et al: Uric acid and chronic kidney disease: which is chasing which? Nephrol Dial Transplant 2013;28:2221–2228.
22 Wu W, Dnyanmote AV, Nigam SK: Remote communication through solute carriers and ATP binding cassette drug transporter pathways: An update on the remote sensing and signaling hypothesis. Mol Pharmacol 2011; 79:795–805.
23 Dalbeth N, et al: Influence of the ABCG2 gout risk 141 K allele on urate metabolism during a fructose challenge. Arthritis Res Ther 2014;16:1–9.
24 Lanaspa MA, et al: Uric acid and fructose: potential biological mechanisms. Semin Nephrol 2011;31:426–432.
25 Nourbakhsh N, Singh P: Role of renal oxygenation and mitochondrial function in the pathophysiology of acute kidney injury. Nephron Clin Pract 2014;127:149–152.
26 Basile DP, Yoder MC: Renal endothelial dysfunction in acute kidney ischemia reperfusion injury. Cardiovasc Hematol Dis Drug Targets 2014;14:3–14.
27 Cristobal-Garcia M, et al: Renal oxidative stress induced by long-term hyperuricemia alters mitochondrial function and maintains systemic hypertension. Oxid Med Cell Longev 2015;2015:535686.
28 Gibbings S, et al: Xanthine oxidoreductase promotes the inflammatory state of mononuclear phagocytes through effects on chemokine expression, peroxisome proliferator-activated receptor-{gamma} sumoylation, and HIF-1{alpha}. J Biol Chem 2011;286: 961–975.
29 Martillo MA, Nazzal L, Crittenden DB: The Crystallization of Monosodium Urate. Curr Rheumatol Rep 2014;16:400.
30 Roncal-Jimenez C, et al: Heat stress nephropathy from exercise-induced uric acid crystalluria: a perspective on mesoamerican nephropathy. Am J Kidney Dis 2016;67:20–30.
31 Rock KL, Kataoka H, Lai JJ: Uric acid as a danger signal in gout and its comorbidities. Nat Rev Rheumatol 2012;9:13–23.
32 Wijkström J, et al: Clinical and pathological characterization of Mesoamerican nephropathy: a new kidney disease in Central America. Am J Kidney Dis 2013;62:908–918.
33 López-Marín L, et al: Histopathology of chronic kidney disease of unknown etiology in Salvadoran agricultural communities. MEDICC Rev 2014;16:49–54.
34 Kupferman J, et al: Characterization of mesoamerican nephropathy in a kidney failure hotspot in nicaragua. Am J Kidney Dis 2016; 68:716–725.
35 Schwarzschild MA, et al: Urate and neuroprotection trials. Lancet Neurol 2014;13:758.

L. Gabriela Sánchez-Lozada, PhD
Laboratory of Renal Physiopathology, Department of Nephrology
Instituto Nacional de Cardiología Ignacio Chávez
Juan Badiano No 1. Sección XVI
14080 Tlalpan, Mexico City (Mexico)
E-Mail lgsanchezlozada@gmail.com

Treviño-Becerra A, Iseki K (eds): Uric Acid in Chronic Kidney Disease.
Contrib Nephrol. Basel, Karger, 2018, vol 192, pp 25–33 (DOI: 10.1159/000484275)

Uric Acid: The Unknown Uremic Toxin

Alejandro Treviño-Becerra
Uremic and Dialysis Clinic, México City, México

Abstract

This review brings together concepts of uric acid metabolism affecting renal parenchyma and its function and the current therapies to reduce hyperuricemia (HyU) and avoid renal disease progression. High uric acid plays an important role in several chronic diseases including kidney diseases such as lithiasis, gout nephropathy, and preeclampsia. In the last 30 years, it has been shown that reducing HyU with low protein and low purine diets in addition to allopurinol creates physiopathological conditions that produce a slight increase in the glomerular filtration rate (GFR). In recent years, in a new era of research in clinical, genetics, pharmacological, and epidemiologic fields, they have been moving forward to support the idea that reduction in HyU could benefit the chronic renal failure (CRF) patients (stage III-IV), thereby avoiding the drop of GFR for undefined mechanisms. There are several clinical trials in progress that show the HyU reducing to very low values and an increased GFR. In a young population, when treating HyU there is a reduction in high blood pressure. There are some reports showing that HyU could play a role in the diabetic nephropathy. Therefore, there have been some speculations that HyU treatment could stop the progression of CRF modifying the natural history of the diseases. So there will be new clinical trials with old and new medication and metabolic procedure to maintain a very low blood levels in the unknown uremic toxin know as uric acid which seems to be the toxin to the damage kidney.

Introduction

This review brings together old concepts of uric acid (UA) metabolism affecting renal parenchyma and its functions, the current therapies to reduce Hyperuricemia (HyU) and avoid renal diseases progression, and some insights to the future HyU therapy.

It is widely known that UA is the final product of the metabolism of purines in humans. Due to the lack of uricase, UA does not unfold into the final particle of metabolism of purines as it does in other animal species; UA in human beings has another substance in the nitrogen pool. Under normal conditions, UA serum values are maintained between 3.0 and 6.0 mg/dL. When there is an altered production or a decrease of excretion of UA, it develops a hyperuricemic syndrome. The most common are gout, tumor lysis, and the presence of urate crystals that can result in renal calculi, and they lead to the chronic nephropathy, a gout nephropathy, renal lithiasis, secondary hypertension, urinary tract infections, and chronic renal failure (CRF) [1, 2].

It has been suggested that UA is one of the causes of chronic kidney disease progression [3–6], and that therapies to lower the UA lead to the reduction of the content of purines in the diet, or pharmacological inhibition of the synthesis of UA, and recently it has been found that therapies are trying to increase UA's discharge by other routes such as the digestive tract [4].

Accumulation of uremic toxins. Toxins are more than 100 in number and some of them play a role in endothelial dysfunction and cardiovascular diseases, possibly in the progression of kidney disease, and are independently associated with mortality. They are investigated in order to search for specific treatments intended to reduce circulating levels of these uremic toxins, such as UA [7]. Recently, a low protein diet has gained importance again because it is a resource for the reduction in the intake of phosphate, purines, and uremic toxins [8].

HyU has 2 sources in CRF. The first one is UA nephropathy that usually occurs with gouty arthritis; the other one is HyU secondary to CRF that results from a decrease of glomerular filtration rate (GFR) below 30 mL/min, in tubular secretion, and an increase in tubular reabsorption; it's been seen as well, leading to a remarkable rise in the level of UA in the blood [5, 6].

HyU is an adverse risk factor in patients with CRF. Studies showed that UA is independently associated with a faster GFR decline. The incidence of renal failure, and even a small increase in the normal range of serum UA may be a risk factor of kidney damage in the population [9–11]. Dialysis may begin later in patients with low weight and small creatinine production because they will develop less metabolic acidosis, hyperkalemia, hyperphosphatemia, and HyU.

Physiopathology

HyU is detrimental to renal function due to [12]:

1. Produces Urates crystal deposits
2. Produces metabolic acidosis
3. Increases renal arterial peripheral resistances

4. Produces endothelial damage
5. Reduces oxidation mechanism
6. Results in High blood pressure
7. Leads to Glomerulosclerosis
8. And all these produces a drop in GFR.

It is known that an increase of UA produces severe vasoconstriction in the renal cortex and arteriopathy. The hemodynamic changes by high UA include the following severe renal vasoconstriction, low renal plasma flow, low GFR and in the isolated nephron, high pre and post glomerular resistances [12].

The mechanism of HyU to cause renal damage is due to oxidative stress and protein glycation, and other mechanisms of renal damage by HyU include several factors despite the low GFR [3]:

1. Renal diseases etiology
2. Metabolic acidosis
3. Hyponatremia
4. Extracellular volume expansion
5. Glomerular hypertension
6. Use of diuretics
7. Diet rich in vegetables
8. Low protein and caloric intake
9. Malnutrition

Chronic Renal Diseases

HyU may be directly pathogenic rather than simply acting as a marker for its associated risk factor. It has been reported that HyU can cause hypertension and that plays a role in the progression of CRF. Several studies have suggested a positive association between HyU and end-stage renal disease, cardiovascular disease and mortality [4, 9, 11–14].

HyU is a common consequence of CRF but may also contribute to CRF progression. In one population-based study, baseline HyU was an independent risk factor for subsequent increase in serum creatinine [15, 16]. A larger study of the same population subsequently identified HyU as an independent risk factor for end-stage renal disease among women but not men. In patients with IgA nephropathy, HyU has emerged as a risk factor for CKD progression [17, 18].

The Tahakata study showed that serum UA concentration was positively associated with renal damage severity suggesting that HyU may be related to glomerular damage in a community-based population. The study shows that HyU is an established risk factor for atherosclerosis and subjects with high serum uric levels have an increased CRF risk. However, it is unknown how UA is related to the development of renal damage in the general population [10].

Bellomo [13], also reported that, in a study of healthy blood donors, the higher the serum UA level, the greater the decline in estimated GFR, with serum UA level being an independent risk factor for renal dysfunction.

Preeclampsia. Further studies define the role of UA in the development of preeclampsia. In the pathogenesis of hypertension, endothelial dysfunction, and renal dysfunction, which are all features of preeclampsia, high plasma levels of UA correlate with disease severity. HyU in preeclampsia was once thought to result solely from reduced renal clearance, but levels of UA also, raise through increased UA production, caused by trophoblast breakdown, cytokine release, and ischemia [19] Monitoring levels of UA is mandatory in the follow-up of these women.

Gout is a highly prevalent comorbidity in patients with CKD and it increases with lower GFR. A third of CKD patients with gout have not reacted to this condition, and among those who are treated, almost half still show HyU. CKD patients represent a high-risk population for gout and screening for treatment of gout, and this population requires special attention [20].

Fructose has been strongly linked with hypertension, HyU, and inflammation. However, the effect of low-fructose diet on inflammation, HyU, and the progression of renal disease has not yet been evaluated in patients with CRF. A slight but not significant reduction in urinary UA and fractional UA excretion was observed while the patients were on the low fructose diet [21]. Fructose is different from other sugars as UA is generated during its metabolism. Serum UA levels have been found to correlate with the intake of fructose and added sugars. Early intervention trials with xanthine oxidase inhibitors such as allopurinol have been found to have benefits on these parameters in both subjects with normal and decreased renal function [8].

More specifically, the usefulness of a low-fructose diet in subjects with CKD could theoretically be unhelpful, given the fact that decreased GFR itself may lead to the retention of UA and sodium, which can cause HyU and hypertension respectively. Excessive intake of fructose, primarily from added sugars, has emerged as a risk factor for HyU, hypertension, metabolic syndrome, and kidney disease. Fructose consumption has markedly increased over the past decades. This intake may increase the urinary excretion of calcium, oxalate, uric acid, and other factors associated with kidney stone risk [12, 14, 21].

Diabetes Mellitus

The in-depth discussion about the HyU role in the prevention or the progression in CRF and the therapeutic action to reduce HyU are still being debated, but a strong interest has recently grown on whether UA or HyU could also be involved in the most frequent nephropathy secondary to D.M. There are several clinical trials and ongoing studies about UA to find out whether the UA has a role in the genesis of the D.M. type I or II or even to test whether HyU is harmful to patients with diabetes and renal failure. There is a great hope that reducing UA is a potential cure for these patients [22–25].

Anti-Hyperuricemic Drugs in Renal Failure

Allopurinol

It has been seen that allopurinol decreases HyU C-reactive protein, slows progression, reduces the risk of cardiovascular events, and has a better impact on residual renal function. Treatment with allopurinol to decrease UA seems useful to restore endothelial function, prevent metabolic acidosis, and slowdown CKF progression. CRF patients (stages II–IV) happen to have a best control of metabolic acidosis and stimulate the endothelial formation when removing HyU [5, 9, 14, 16].

Among 54 patients with CKD, the randomized group with allopurinol treatment showed stable serum creatinine values over 12 months, whereas patients in the control group showed an increase, but this benefit did not correlate with UA levels. Possible mechanisms whereby HyU may contribute to CRF progression are glomerular hypertension, endothelial dysfunction, and proinflammatory effects [6].

Why is allopurinol so effective [26, 27]?

1. Leads to reduction of urates levels
2. Results in inhibition of enzyme oxidase
3. Other mechanisms that make allopurinol effective are under investigation.

The available evidence evaluating the safety and efficacy of allopurinol as a renoprotective agent in patients with CKD is limited to a small number of single-center studies. Nevertheless, given that there is abundant evidence of an association between UA and CKD progression from epidemiological and animal studies, UA-lowering therapy may retard the progression of CKD [6, 15].

In the case of patients with reduced kidney function, allopurinol therapy may be associated with adverse reactions more frequently and may cause prolonged hypouricemia. Allopurinol can cause liver dysfunction. The incidence of side effects is high (4%), and severe adverse reactions such as hypersensitivity reaction (including Stevens-Johnson Syndrome), agranulocytosis, and hypersensitivity, vasculitis may occur [28].

Topiroxostat is a selective inhibitor of xanthine oxidase; it is effective in reducing serum urate level in HyU patients with or without gout. A dosage of Topiroxostat 60 mg effectively reduced the serum urate level in the hyperuricemic stage III chronic kidney disease patients with or without gout [29].

Febuxostat. A new, non-purine, selective inhibitor of xanthine oxidase, is metabolized mainly by glucuronidation and oxidation in the liver. It is excreted by both urinary and fecal pathways, and could be well tolerated and effective in CKD patients with mild to moderate renal dysfunction without dose reduction. Some clinical studies have shown that febuxostat has a more potent UA-lowering effect than conventional therapy with allopurinol [30, 31].

Among the mechanisms that are involved in the beneficial effects of a better control of serum UA with respect to changes of GFR, febuxostat reduced serum UA levels more effectively than conventional therapy and might have a renoprotective effect in HyU patients with CKD.

Febuxostat exerted a reliable and stable clinical effect that was so far greater than allopurinol and other conventional treatments in reducing serum UA in CKD patients with HyU. Results suggest that the renoprotective effect of febuxostat might be independent of an effect on serum UA reduction and hypertension, such as reduction of plasma rennin activity, inhibition of oxidative stress, and improvement of endothelial dysfunction. The results demonstrated that compared to conventional treatment, febuxostat exerted a more stable and reliable action in reducing serum UA levels. It also showed a renoprotective effect, improving levels of urinary protein, urinary albumin, and tubulointerstial markers [31].

However, few data are available regarding the clinical effect of febuxostat in patients with CKD. Notably, the evidentiary basis for the safety and efficacy of uric acid-lowering therapy for preventing CKD progression is scant and additional large-scale trials are now needed [31].

To treat HyU, other medications as Losartan [32], empagliflozin, [33] and even probiotics [34] have been used. But the results are less consistent than the results obtained with the use of xanthine oxidase drugs.

Clinical Experiences

In a period when we did not have access to chronic dialysis treatments, it was common practice to have CRF patients with urea at levels of 400–600 mg% or more, creatinine at 18–20 mg%, and UA above 12 mg% or more. We called this condition secondary HyU and no attention was given to diminish it.

Thirty years ago, I initiated a series of clinical trails to counteract HyU in CRF by reducing the amount of dietary proteins and purines, and prescribing high allopurinol doses (10 mg/kg of body weight). The results have been an increase in urine production, the normalization of blood UA levels, the concomitant 20–25% reduction in blood urea, and 15–20 increase in the GFR for periods of up to 3 months to 6 years [3, 15].

Afterwards, the therapeutic action was to diminish purines from the diet or completely eliminate vegetable and animal sources with an isocaloric diet with normal fluid intake, and to give allopurinol at high doses. Allopurinol toxicity was not observed with these high doses. Consequently, the most used doses had been 10 mg/kg of body weight and in some cases, it is reduced to 5mg/kg. One study followed 60 patients for a period of 5 years. We observed UA reduction, decrease of blood urea, and an increase in GFR. A 25% reduction in UA from 6.4 ± 2.3 to 4.2 ± 1.4 resulted in an increase in the GFR from 20.3 ± 7.4 to 24.2 ± 8.2 mL/min (15%) and urea decreases from 101 ± 30 to 86 ± 27 mg% (15%). The subgroup was called "poor responded" probably called like that because it did not follow a correct diet or due to genetic factors. There is a group of CRF patients (stage IV) receiving this treatment that keeps a stable GFR for many years.

In another communication, it was observed that in individuals with unilateral nephrectomy for renal adenocarcinoma, after 2 weeks of free purine diet and allopurinol, there was an increase in the renal plasma flow by 25% and the effect was maintained during the 6 months follow-up [35].

From all these experiences, it was observed that as soon the UA decreased to low serum values, patients experienced a feeling of well-being, with a reduction of anorexia and digestive symptoms and complete elimination of asthenia. Patients consequently eat and feel better and they are more cooperative. It is possible to ameliorate the uremic state and preserve renal function. The control of HyU is a simple therapeutic maneuver and is the priority treatment plan in CRF patients [3].

Conclusion

It is necessary to avoid the hyperuricemic state in CRF. The HyU control by diet and drugs in patients with progressive renal failure is a simple and easy therapeutic maneuver to ameliorate uremic symptoms and to diminish the drop in GFR. This therapy is extremely useful in CRF patients. More clinical and physiopathological research is needed in the future in order to have a definitive answer and clear the air whether uric acid is the unknown uremic toxin.

References

1 Johnson RJ, Kivlighn SD, Kim YG, et al: Reappraisal of the pathogenesis and consequences of hyperuricemia in hypertension, cardiovascular disease, and renal disease. Am J Kidney Dis 1999;33:225–234.

2 Taal MW, Brenner BM: Predicting initiation and progression of chronic kidney disease: developing renal risk scores. Kidney int 2006; 70:21694–1705.

3 Treviño BA, Cuevas SRM, Velazquez RJ: Dietas bajas en purinas, mantienen al año la filtración glomerular en insuficiencia renal moderada. Gaceta Médica de México 1989; 125:271–278.

4 Kang DH, Nakagawa T, Feng L, et al: A role for uric acid in the progression of renal disease. J Am Soc Nephrol 2002;13:2888–2897.

5 Johnson RJ, Kang DH, Feig D, et al: Is there a pathogenetic role for uric acid in hypertension and cardiovascular and renal disease? Hypertension 2003;41:1183–1190.

6 Iseki K, Ikemiya Y, Inoue T, et al: Significance of hyperuricemia as a risk factor for developing ESRD in a screened cohort. Am J Kidney Dis 2004;44:642–650.

7 Vanholder R, De Smet R, Glorieux G, et.al: Review on uremic toxins: classification, concentration, and interindividual variability. Kidney Int 2003;63:1934–1943.

8 Johnson EJ, Rideous BA: Uric acid and diet: insight into the epidemic of cardiovascular disease. N Eng J Med 2004;1071–1073.

9 Mok Y, Lee SJ, Kim MS, Cui W, Moon MY, Jee SH: Serum uric acid and chronic kidney disease: the Severance cohort study. Nephrol Dial Transplant 2012;27:1831–1835.

10 Suzuki K, Konta T, Kudo K, Sato H, Ikeda A, Ichikawa K, Ueno Y, Kato T, Kayama T, Kubota I: The association between serum uric acid and renal damage in a community based population. Clin Exp Nephrol 2013;17:541–548.

11 Goicoechea M, de Vinuesa SG, Verdalles U, et al: Effect of allopurinol in chronic kidney disease progression and cardiovascular visk. Clin J Am Soc Nephrol 2010;5:1388–1393.

12 Madero M, Sarnak MJ, Wang X et al: Uric acid and long-term outcomes in CKD. Am J Kidney Dis 2009;53:796–803.

13 Bellomo G: Uric acid and chronic kidney disease. A time to act? World J Nephrol 2013;2: 17–25.

14 Johnson RJ, Nakagawa J, Jalal D, Sanchéz-lozada LG, Kang DH, Ritz E: Uric/acid and chronic kidney disease: which is chasing which? Nephrol Dial Trasplant 2013;28: 2221–2228.

15 Treviño BA, Recinos MG, Velazquez RJ: Orally induced uremic detoxification by low purine and phosphate diet and high doses of allopurinol and aluminium hydroxide. In: Giordano C, Friedman C, De Santo E, Meyer M, (eds). Prevention of Progressive Uremia, vol. II. Field and Wood Medical Publ., New York, NY, USA, 1989.

16 Johnson RJ, Kivlighn SD, Kim YG, Suga S, Fogo AB: Reappraisal of the pathogenesis and consequences of hyperuricemia in hypertelnsion cardiovascular disease and renal disease. Am J Kidney Dis 1999;33:225–234.

17 Hsu CY, Iribarren C, McCulloch CE, et al: Risk factors for end-stage renal disease: 25-years follow-up. Arch Intern Med 2009; 342–250.

18 Treviño-Becerra A: Hipotrigliceridemia and hyperuricemia in IgA nephropathy. Nephro Dial Transplant 2011;16:639–643.

19 Martin AC, Brown MA: Could uric acid have a pathogenic role in pre-eclampsia? Nat Rev Nephrol 2010;6:744–748.

20 Jing J, Kielstein JT, Schultheiss UT, Sitter T, Titze SI, et al; GCKD Study Investigators: Prevalence and correlates of gout in a large cohort of patients with chronic kidney disease: the German Chronic Kidney Disease (GCKD) Study. Nephrol Dial Transplant 2015;30:613–621.

21 Brymora A, Flisinski M, Johnson RJ, Goszka G, Stefariska A, Manititus J: Low-fructose diet lowers blood pressure and inflammation in patients with chronic kidney disease. Nephrol. Dial Transplant 2012;27:608–612.

22 Zoppini G, Targher G, Chonchol M, Ortalda V, Abaterusso C, Pichiri I, Negri C, Bonora E: Serum uric acid levels and incident chronic kidney disease in patients with Type 2 diabetes and preserved kidney function. Diabetes Care 2012;35:99–104.

23 Ahola AJ, Sandholm N, Forsblom C, et al: The serum uric acid concentration is not causally linked to diabetic nephropathy in type 1 diabetes. Kidney Int 2017;91:1178–1185.

24 Ficociello LH, Rosolowsky ET, Niewczas MA, et al: High-normal serum uric acid increases risk of early progressive renal function loss in type 1 diabetes: results of a 6-year follow-up. Diabetes Care 2010;33:1337–1343.
25 Maahs DM, Caramori L, Cherney DZ, Galecki AT, Gao C, Jalal D, Perkins BA, Pop-Busui R, Rossing P, Mauer M, Doria A; PERL Consortium: Uric acid lowering to prevent kidney function loss in diabetes: the preventing early renal function loss (PERL) allopurinol study. Curr Diab Rep 2013;13:550–559.
26 Bose B, Badve VS, Hiremath SS, Boudville N, Brown FG, Cass A, et al: Effects of uric acid-lowering therapy on renal outcomes: a systematic review and meta-analysis. Nephrol Dial Transplant 2014;29:406–413.
27 Siu YP, Leung KT, Tong MK, Kwan TH: Use of allopurinol in slowing the progression of renal disease through its ability to lower serum uric acid level. Am J Kidney Dis 2006;47: 51–59.
28 Chan SH, Tan T: HLA and allopurinol drug eruption. Dermatologica 1989;17.32–33.
29 Hosoya T, Ohno I, Nomura S, Hisatome I, Uchida S, Fujimori S, Yamamoto T, Hara S: Effects of topiroxostat on the serum urate levels and urinary albumin excretion in hyperuricemic stage 3 chronic kidney disease patients with or without gout. Clin Exp Nephrol 2014;18:876–884.
30 Tanaka K, Nakayama M, Kanno K, Kimura H, Watanabe K, et al: Renoprotective effects of febuxostat in hyperuricemic patients with chronic kidney disease: a parallel-group, randomized, controlled trial. Clin Exp Nephrol 2015;19:1044–1053.
31 Naoyuki K, Shin F, Toshikazu H, et al: An allopurinol-controlled, multicenter, randomized, open-label, parallel between-group, comparative study of febuxostat (TMX-67), a non-purine-selective inhibitor of xanthine oxidase, in patients with hyperuricemia including those with gout in Japan: phase 2 exploratory clinical study. J Clinic Rheumatol 2211;17:544–549.
32 Miao Y, Ottenbros SA, Laverman GD, Brenner BM, Cooper ME, Parving HH, Grobbee DE, Shahinfar S, de Zeeuw D, Lambers Heerspink HJ: Effect of a reduction in uric acid on renal outcomes during losartan treatment: a post hoc analysis ofthe rof endpoints in n-insulin-dependent diabetes mellitus with the angiotensin II antagonist losartan trial. Hypertension 2011;58:22–27.
33 Wanner C, lnzucchi SE, Lachin JM, Fitchett D, von Eynatten M, Mattheus M, Johansen OE, Woerle HJ, BroedL UC, Zinman B; EMPA-REG Outcome Investigators: Empagliflozin and progression of kidney disease in type 2 diabetes. N Engl J Med 2016;375:323–334.
34 Ranganathan N, Pechenyak B, Vyas U, Ranganathan P, DeLoach S, Falkner B, Weinberg A, Saggi SJ, Friedman DI: Dose escalation, safety and impact of a Strain-specific probiOtic (renadyl) on stages III and IV chronic kidney disease patients. J Nephrol Therapeut 2013;3:141.
35 Treviño BA, Trinidad RP, Muñoz R, Sandoval R, Mondragon L: Modifications of Renal Plasmatic Flow in Patients with unilateral nephrectomy who receivel a diet without purines Abstract. 74, Int Symposium of Hemoperfusion. Rostock GDR 1988.

Alejandro Treviño-Becerra
Uremic and Dialysis Clinic
Tuxpan 16-104 Col. Roma
06760 México City (México)
E-Mail atreve16@yahoo.com.mx

Treviño-Becerra A, Iseki K (eds): Uric Acid in Chronic Kidney Disease.
Contrib Nephrol. Basel, Karger, 2018, vol 192, pp 34–40 (DOI: 10.1159/000484276)

The Association between Serum Uric Acid and Renal Damage: The Takahata Study – New Insights

Tsuneo Konta[a] · Keita Kamei[a] · Kazunobu Ichikawa[a] · Takamasa Kayama[b] · Isao Kubota[a]

[a]Department of Cardiology, Pulmonology, and Nephrology, and [b]Global COE, Yamagata University School of Medicine, Yamagata, Japan

Abstract

Background: Hyperuricemia is a risk factor for causing end-stage kidney disease and cardiovascular disease in the general population; however, several aspects, such as the site of kidney damaged by hyperuricemia and the threshold levels of serum uric acid for the development of renal damage, have not been fully clarified. ***Summary:*** To examine these aspects, we analyzed data from the Takahata study, a community-based cohort study involving participants of an annual health check-up, and used urinary albumin creatinine ratio (UACR) and urinary β2-microglobulin creatinine ratio (UBCR) in spot urine as indices of glomerular and tubular damage respectively. In cross-sectional analysis, increased serum uric acid levels were accompanied by higher UACR values and lower UBCR values. Multivariate analysis revealed that albuminuria (UACR ≥30 mg/g), but not elevated UBCR, was independently associated with increased uric acid (≥7 mg/dL for males, ≥6 mg/dL for females). In longitudinal analysis, uric acid at baseline was an independent factor for a 1-year increase in the UACR. Cox-proportional hazard model analysis with adjustment for possible confounders including age, renal function, and comorbidities revealed that hyperuricemia was an independent risk factor for all-cause and cardiovascular mortality in females. ***Key Messages:*** Our results revealed that elevated uric acid is an independent risk factor for glomerular damage, but not tubular damage, and that the risk for renal damage and mortality might be increased at the high-normal range of uric acid in the community-based population.

Introduction

Previous studies have shown that hyperuricemia increases the risk for cardiovascular disease, premature death [1, 2], and incidental chronic kidney disease (CKD) [3]. However, conflicting results have been reported in other studies. In the general population, increased uric acid levels were independently associated with end-stage kidney disease in women, but not in men [4]. In a meta-analysis, elevated serum uric acid levels were shown to significantly increase the risk of all-cause mortality in men, but not in women [5]. In patients with CKD, hyperuricemia was found to be a risk for all-cause and CVD mortality, but not for kidney failure [6]. In the elderly, uric acid levels show a significant but weak association with the progression of kidney disease [7]. Furthermore, one report documented that the risk for end-stage kidney disease was increased at different threshold values for men (≥7 mg/dL) and women (≥6 mg/dL) [4]. Therefore, the association between an increase in serum uric acid and kidney disease is still up for debate. In particular, aspects, such as the site of kidney damaged by hyperuricemia and the threshold levels of serum uric acid for the development of renal damage, have not been fully clarified in the community-based population.

The Takahata Study

To address these points, we analyzed data from the Takahata study, a community-based cohort study [8]. The Takahata study is a part of the ongoing Molecular Epidemiological Study involving participants of an annual health check-up, to which all inhabitants over 40 years of age in Takahata, Japan were invited. In this study, we used the urinary excretion of albumin and β2-microglobulin in spot urine as markers of glomerular and tubular damage (urinary albumin creatinine ratio [UACR] and urinary β2-microglobulin creatinine ratio [UBCR], respectively). The study population for this analysis included 3,126 subjects (1,393 males, 1,733 females, mean age 62) without renal insufficiency (estimated glomerular filtration rate <60 mL/min/1.73 m^2) or a previous history of gout or kidney disease. The mean serum uric acid (mg/dL) was 5.8 ± 1.3 (SD) in men and 4.5 ± 1.1 in women. Hyperuricemia (≥7 mg/dL) was detected in 245 subjects (7.8%) out of the total population (214 men [15.4%], 31 women [1.8%]).

Renal Tubular Damage and Uric Acid

Severe and prolonged hyperuricemia is often accompanied by tubulointerstitial nephritis via the formation of uric acid crystals, that is, so-called gouty kidney. Therefore, it was expected that an increase in serum uric acid would be associated with renal tubular damages in this community-based population. Surprisingly, a cross-sectional analysis using the baseline data of serum uric acid and

UBCR revealed that in men, UBCR values and the prevalence of high UBCR (≥300 μg/g) decreased along with increases in uric acid, whereas in women, the UBCR values decreased along with increases in uric acid. However, the prevalence of high UBCR was not significantly related to uric acid levels. Further, in order to investigate the independent association between uric acid and UBCR, we performed a multivariate logistic regression analysis including confounding factors such as age, hypertension, diabetes, hypercholesterolemia, urinary sodium excretion, obesity, alcohol consumption, and estimated glomerular filtration rate. UBCR was found to be negatively associated with uric acid in men, but not in women. These results suggest that increased serum uric acid levels were unlikely to be a cause of renal tubular damage in this population.

Glomerular Damage and Uric Acid

Next, to examine the relationship between serum uric acid levels and glomerular damage, we used albuminuria (UACR ≥30 mg/g) as a marker of glomerular damage. In a cross-sectional analysis, increased UACR values and the prevalence of albuminuria were associated with elevated uric acid levels in women. In men, the UACR values were associated with increased uric acid, but the increase in the prevalence of albuminuria was not significant. In multivariate logistic regression analysis, in both men and women, albuminuria was independently related to increased uric acid levels after adjustment for possible confounders, especially in the uric acid ranges of ≥7 mg/dL in men and ≥6 mg/dL in women.

Additionally, in order to investigate the potential effect of serum uric acid on the progression of albuminuria, we longitudinally examined the 1-year changes in UACR based on basal uric acid levels. In both men and women, 1-year UACR changes showed a significant positive association with baseline uric acid levels. The multivariate linear regression analysis with adjustment for possible confounders showed that uric acid at baseline was an independent factor for 1-year changes in UACR. This result suggests the significance of uric acid as an aggravating factor for albuminuria and glomerular damage. In patients with hyperuricemia, glomerular lesions are less obvious and are typically considered secondary changes due to tubulointerstitial damage or concomitant diseases such as hypertension and obesity. However, our finding implies that hyperuricemia may directly provoke glomerular injury.

Based on the observed association between the UACR and UBCR values and serum uric acid levels, it can be speculated that the site of kidney damage due to increased serum uric acid is mainly the glomerular vessels, rather than the tubulointerstitial lesion in the community-based population.

Uric Acid Threshold Levels for the Development of Renal Damage

Currently, one basic definition of hyperuricemia (>7 mg/dL) is applied to both men and women. This threshold value is based on the observation that the level of uric acid at which the crystallization of uric acid occurs is >7 mg/dL in the blood. Notably, the Takahata study showed that an increase in UACR levels and prevalence of albuminuria were observed in men with uric acid ≥7 mg/dL and women with uric acid ≥6 mg/dL. This suggests that the threshold levels for serum uric acid to inflict glomerular damage differ according to gender (lower in women than in men). Iseki et al. [4] documented that gender-specific threshold levels of serum uric acid (7 mg/dL uric acid in men and 6 mg/dL in women) are an independent predictor of incident CKD. In a nationwide large cohort including 165,847 community-based subjects, we showed that the odds ratio for incidental renal insufficiency was significantly increased with uric acid levels of ≥6.3 mg/dL in males and ≥5.5 mg/dL in females [9]. This is in accordance with previous reports in which cardiovascular mortality in females was shown to increase with serum uric acid levels of ≥5.5 mg/dL [1] and in which the association between time-varying serum uric acid and increased cardiovascular risk tended to be stronger in women than in men [10]. These findings suggest that the risk for the development and the progression of renal damage and cardiovascular disease might be increased at a slightly elevated level of serum uric acid, even within the normal range. Moreover, the threshold values of uric acid might be lower in women than in men.

The reason why the threshold levels of uric acid for renal and cardiovascular diseases are lower in women than in men is unknown. One possible explanation pertains to the effect of sex hormones on the metabolism of uric acid. Estrogenic compounds enhance renal urate excretion [11] and keep serum uric acid levels lower in females than in males. The estrogenic compounds are also known to have a vascular protective property. Therefore, it is speculated that the increase in uric acid in females is induced by a combination of decreased protective estrogenic compounds and uric acid overproduction, which might intensify the effect of uric acid on renal function in females.

The Mechanism by Which Uric Acid Causes Renal Damage

The mechanism by which uric acid induces renal damage has not yet been fully elucidated. In gouty kidney, the deposition of uric acid crystals causes renal tubulointerstitial damage. However, such typical gouty changes are rarely observed in renal biopsy specimens in subjects with hyperuricemia and reduced renal function. In recent years, a series of experimental and clinical studies have suggested that uric acid can cause tissue injury, irrespective of the formation of uric acid crystals. One study demonstrated that the oxidative stress induced by the metabolism of uric acid impairs vascular endothelial cells [12]. Other studies described that uric acid is directly absorbed into the vascular endothelium and vascular smooth muscle by URAT1, a urate transporter [13], and that it induces inflammation of vessel walls, promoting arterial sclerosis [14]. It has also been reported that uric acid is produced by xanthine oxidase and hypoxanthine under ischemic conditions and that it directly stimulates vascular smooth muscle cell proliferation in vitro [15]. In rats, hyperuricemia was shown to induce not only systemic hypertension, but also glomerular hypertension [16]. Moreover, mild hyperuricemia induces the arteriolopathy of preglomerular vessels, which impairs the autoregulatory response of afferent arterioles, resulting in glomerular hypertension [17]. Clinically, serum uric acid is associated with microalbuminuria and subclinical atherosclerosis in men with type 2 diabetes mellitus [18] and arteriosclerosis in renal biopsy specimens [19].

According to these findings, renal damage may be caused by a mechanism similar to the systemic effect of uric acid that directly impairs the vascular system (intrarenal arteries of various sizes including the glomerulus). If a mechanism that does not involve the formation of uric acid crystals is implicated in renal damage in the community-based population, it is possible that renal injury may become significant at a high-normal value of uric acid.

The Link between Uric Acid, Renal Damage, and Mortality

In addition to the association between uric acid and albuminuria, the Takahata study demonstrated the association between serum uric acid, renal damage, and mortality. Albuminuria was shown to be a strong predictor of all-cause and cardiovascular mortality, the significance of which was maintained after adjusting for possible confounders [20]. Furthermore, increased serum uric acid levels were independently associated with cardiovascular death, especially in women [21]. The findings from the Takahata study suggest that increases of uric acid within the normal range might induce vascular damage, including glomerular damage, and shed new light on the link between uric acid, renal damage, cardiovascular disease, and mortality in the community-based population (Fig. 1).

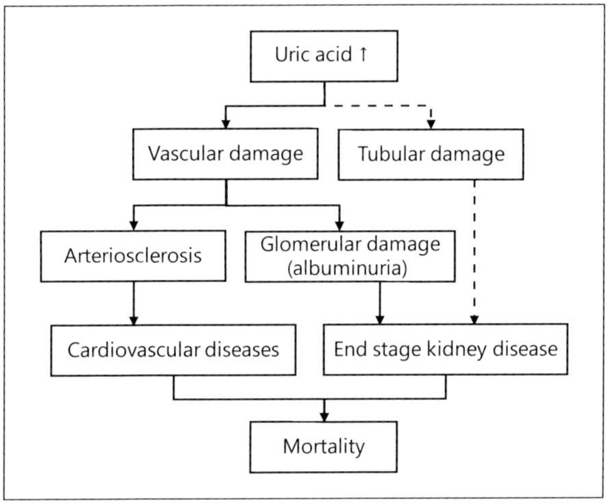

Fig. 1. The association between uric acid, renal damage, and mortality in community-based population.

Conclusion

In conclusion, the Takahata study showed that increased uric acid is an independent risk factor for glomerular damage, but not tubular damage, and that the renal damage might develop in the context of the high-normal range of uric acid. Further studies are necessary to determine the optimal values of serum uric acid for the prevention and treatment of renal and cardiovascular diseases.

References

1 Fang J, Alderman MH: Serum uric acid and cardiovascular mortality the NHANES I epidemiologic follow-up study, 1971–1992. National Health and Nutrition Examination Survey. JAMA 2000;283:2404–2410.

2 Chen JH, Chuang SY, Chen HJ, Yeh WT, Pan WH: Serum uric acid level as an independent risk factor for all-cause, cardiovascular, and ischemic stroke mortality: a Chinese cohort study. Arthr Rheum 2009;61:225–232.

3 Iseki K, Oshiro S, Tozawa M, Iseki C, Ikemiya Y, Takishita S: Significance of hyperuricemia on the early detection of renal failure in a cohort of screened subjects. Hypertens Res 2001;24:691–697.

4 Iseki K, Ikemiya Y, Inoue T, Iseki C, Kinjo K, Takishita S: Significance of hyperuricemia as a risk factor for developing ESRD in a screened cohort. Am J Kidney Dis 2004;44: 642–650.

5 Zhao G, Huang L, Song M, Song Y: Baseline serum uric acid level as a predictor of cardiovascular disease related mortality and all-cause mortality: a meta-analysis of prospective studies. Atherosclerosis 2013;231:61–68.

6 Madero M, Sarnak MJ, Wang X, Greene T, Beck GJ, Kusek JW, Collins AJ, Levey AS, Menon V: Uric acid and long-term outcomes in CKD. Am J Kidney Dis 2009;53:796–803.

7 Chonchol M, Shlipak MG, Katz R, Sarnak MJ, Newman AB, Siscovick DS, Kestenbaum B, Carney JK, Fried LF: Relationship of uric acid with progression of kidney disease. Am J Kidney Dis 2007;50:239–247.

8 Suzuki K, Konta T, Kudo K, Sato H, Ikeda A, Ichikawa K, Ueno Y, Kato T, Kayama T, Kubota I: The association between serum uric acid and renal damage in a community-based population: the Takahata study. Clin Exp Nephrol 2013;17:541–548.

9 Kamei K, Konta T, Hirayama A, Suzuki K, Ichikawa K, Fujimoto S, Iseki K, Moriyama T, Yamagata K, Tsuruya K, Kimura K, Narita I, Kondo M, Asahi K, Watanabe T: A slight increase within the normal range of serum uric acid and the decline in renal function: associations in a community-based population. Nephrol Dial Transplant 2014;29:2286–2292.
10 Høieggen A, Alderman MH, Kjeldsen SE, Julius S, Devereux RB, De Faire U, Fyhrquist F, Ibsen H, Kristianson K, Lederballe-Pedersen O, Lindholm LH, Nieminen MS, Omvik P, Oparil S, Wedel H, Chen C, Dahlöf B; LIFE Study Group: The impact of serum uric acid on cardiovascular outcomes in the LIFE study. Kidney Int 2004;65:1041–1049.
11 Antón FM, García Puig J, Ramos T, González P, Ordás J: Sex differences in uric acid metabolism in adults: evidence for a lack of influence of estradiol-17 beta (E2) on the renal handling of urate. Metabolism 1986;35:343–348.
12 Kang DH, Park SK, Lee IK, Johnson RJ: Uric acid-induced C-reactive protein expression: implication on cell proliferation and nitric oxide production of human vascular cells. J Am Soc Nephrol 2005;16:3553–3562.
13 Price KL, Sautin YY, Long DA, Zhang L, Miyazaki H, Mu W, Endou H, Johnson RJ: Human vascular smooth muscle cells express a urate transporter. J Am Soc Nephrol 2006;17:1791–1795.
14 Johnson RJ, Kang DH, Feig D, Kivlighn S, Kanellis J, Watanabe S, Tuttle KR, Rodriguez-Iturbe B, Herrera-Acosta J, Mazzali M: Is there a pathogenetic role for uric acid in hypertension and cardiovascular and renal disease? Hypertension 2003;41:1183–1190.
15 Mazzali M, Kanellis J, Han L, Feng L, Xia YY, Chen Q, Kang DH, Gordon KL, Watanabe S, Nakagawa T, Lan HY, Johnson RJ: Hyperuricemia induces a primary renal arteriolopathy in rats by a blood pressure-independent mechanism. Am J Physiol Renal Physiol 2002;282:F991–F997.
16 Mazzali M, Hughes J, Kim YG, Jefferson JA, Kang DH, Gordon KL, Lan HY, Kivlighn S, Johnson RJ: Elevated uric acid increases blood pressure in the rat by a novel crystal-independent mechanism. Hypertension 2001;38:1101–1106.
17 Sánchez-Lozada LG, Tapia E, Santamaría J, Avila-Casado C, Soto V, Nepomuceno T, Rodríguez-Iturbe B, Johnson RJ, Herrera-Acosta J: Mild hyperuricemia induces vasoconstriction and maintains glomerular hypertension in normal and remnant kidney rats. Kidney Int 2005;67:237–247.
18 Fukui M, Tanaka M, Shiraishi E, Harusato I, Hosoda H, Asano M, Kadono M, Hasegawa G, Yoshikawa T, Nakamura N: Serum uric acid is associated with microalbuminuria and subclinical atherosclerosis in men with type 2 diabetes mellitus. Metabolism 2008;57:625–629.
19 Kohagura K, Kochi M, Miyagi T, Kinjyo T, Maehara Y, Nagahama K, Sakima A, Iseki K, Ohya Y: An association between uric acid levels and renal arteriolopathy in chronic kidney disease: a biopsy-based study. Hypertens Res 2013;36:43–49.
20 Konta T, Kudo K, Sato H, Ichikawa K, Ikeda A, Suzuki K, Hirayama A, Shibata Y, Watanabe T, Daimon M, Kato T, Ueno Y, Kayama T, Kubota I: Albuminuria is an independent predictor of all-cause and cardiovascular mortality in the Japanese population: the Takahata study. Clin Exp Nephrol 2013;17:805–810.
21 Kamei K, Konta T, Ichikawa K, Sato H, Suzuki N, Kabasawa A, Suzuki K, Hirayama A, Shibata Y, Watanabe T, Kato T, Ueno Y, Kayama T, Kubota I: Serum uric acid levels and mortality in the Japanese population: the Yamagata (Takahata) study. Clin Exp Nephrol 2016;20:904–909.

Dr. Tsuneo Konta
Department of Cardiology, Pulmonology, and Nephrology
Yamagata University School of Medicine
2-2-2, Iida-Nishi
Yamagata 990-9585 (Japan)
E-Mail kkonta@med.id.yamagata-u.ac.jp

Treviño-Becerra A, Iseki K (eds): Uric Acid in Chronic Kidney Disease.
Contrib Nephrol. Basel, Karger, 2018, vol 192, pp 41–47 (DOI: 10.1159/000484277)

Significance of Hyperuricemia among Community-Based Screening Participants

Kunitoshi Iseki

Clinical Research Support Center, Tomishiro Central Hospital, Okinawa, Japan

Abstract

Background: Chronic kidney disease (CKD) is a risk factor of cardiovascular disease (CVD) and end-stage renal disease (ESRD). Early detection and management of risk factors of incidence and progression of CKD are necessary. We have been studying these risk factors among community-based screening participants in Okinawa, Japan. Okinawa was one of the longevity areas in the world; however, the incidence and prevalence of ESRD increased. In Japan, the incidence of ESRD is 2 times higher in men compared to that in women. Such gender difference in ESRD incidence may be explained by the difference in lifestyle-related factors such as obesity and metabolic syndrome. ***Summary:*** We have shown the significance of hyperuricemia on the incidence of ESRD and progression of CKD. Hyperuricemia was associated with increased risk of developing ESRD, in particular women. Although the causal relationship between the levels of serum uric acid (SUA) and changes in estimated glomerular filtration rate (eGFR) was not clear, we observed that high SUA was associated with larger decrease in eGFR. People with hyperuricemia, >7.0 mg/dL, may have an unhealthy lifestyle. We observed to see if intensive care, involving regular monitoring of body mass index and lifestyle and intervention when appropriate by dietitians and general practitioners, led to improved renal outcomes among patients with stage 3 CKD, compared to standard care. The benefit was observed in patients with CKD stage 3b. ***Key Message:*** Hyperuricemia is closely associated with the incidence and progression of CKD. Lifestyle modification including hyperuricemia would be the basis of management of CKD patients.

Introduction

Social and economic burden due to chronic kidney disease (CKD) is becoming a major problem not only in developed but also in developing countries. CKD is the cause of end-stage renal disease (ESRD) requiring renal replacement therapy and cardiovascular disease (CVD). Therefore, early detection and management of CKD is warranted. In Japan, a general health screening program has been adopted for more than 40 years. We have been studying the outcomes mainly the incidence of ESRD among the screened subjects in Okinawa, Japan [1, 2]. We are also studying the mortality risk using nationwide screening cohort [3].

In Japan, the incidence and prevalence of ESRD are still increasing, particularly in men (Fig. 1). Reasons are not clear, however; the impact of lifestyle changes with high prevalence of metabolic syndrome and obesity may explain these trends. Hyperuricemia is also common in men than in women (Fig. 2). Hyperuricemia could be a marker for unhealthy lifestyle involving smoking, being overweight, large alcohol intake, less physical activity, and erratic eating habits.

In this paper, epidemiological studies concerning the role of hyperuricemia in CKD, which were conducted in Okinawa and other parts of Japan in the past 20 years are summarized.

Epidemiological Studies

Among the laboratory variables commonly measured in general screening, dipstick proteinuria, serum creatinine (automatically calculated estimated glomerular filtration rate [eGFR]), blood pressure, and fasting blood glucose (diabetes mellitus) are strong predictors of ESRD. In addition to these variables, we reported the significance of hyperuricemia on the incidence of CKD [4, 5] and ESRD [6, 7]. In women, the risk of developing ESRD was significantly elevated at serum uric acid (SUA) 6.0 mg/dL.

We also observed the close relationship between hyperuricemia and CVD risk [8], hypertension [9], metabolic syndrome [10, 11], and renal arteriopathy in biopsy specimen [12].

Outside Okinawa, a similar relationship between SUA and CKD has been reported [13, 14]. However, the incidence of CKD may differ by using estimating GFR, particularly in relatively young adults [14]. Changes in eGFR may not necessarily be linear. SUA is a factor predicting eGFR decline by a within-patient analysis for time-varying risk factors of CKD progression [4, 15]. In type 1 DM, higher the SUA the risk of rapid decline in eGFR increased [16].

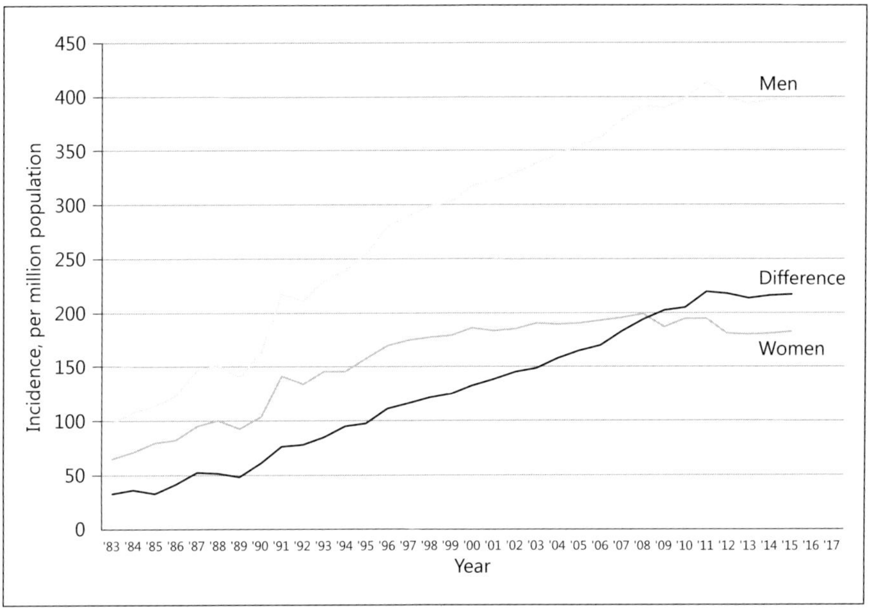

Fig. 1. Incidence of ESRD by gender in Japan (Data are from the Annual Report of the Japanese Society for Dialysis Therapy 1983–2015).

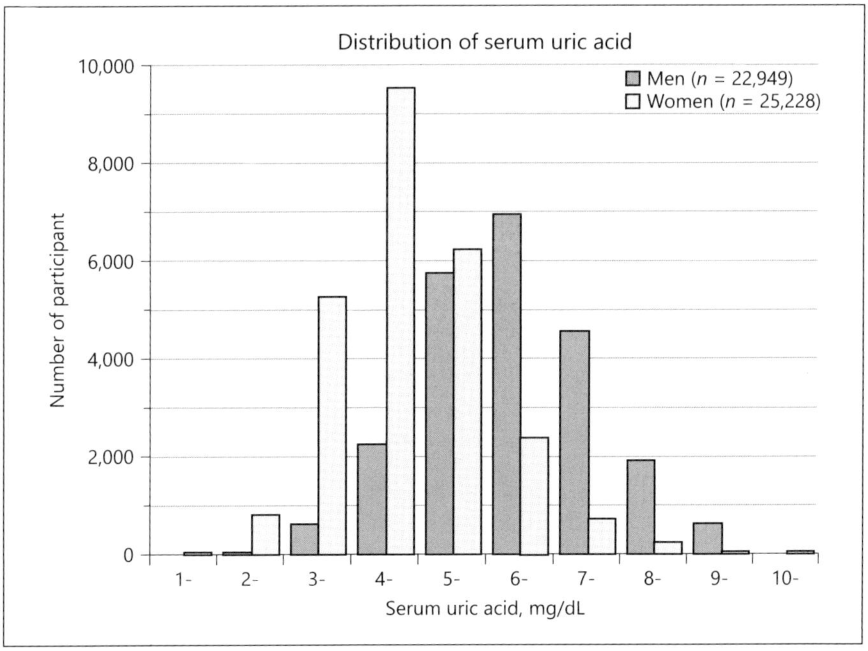

Fig. 2. Distribution of serum uric acid among participants in general screening in Okinawa (cited from ref. [7]).

According to the nationwide cohort, SUA was shown to be associated with the incidence of nonfatal stroke [17]. This observation was confirmed in Takahata study, as hyperuricemia was an independent risk for all-cause and CVD mortality in female [18]. Also, in a representative Japanese general population, UA level was significantly associated with atrial fibrillation, independently of other cardiovascular risk factors [19]. Interestingly, the threshold SUA level was different between men (≥5.4 mg/dL) and women (≥5.0 mg/dL).

Hara et al. [20] reported the longitudinal changes in urine pH and SUA. SUA is increasing gradually both in men and women, as the urine pH declined. Such observation may reflect the increase in obesity and metabolic syndrome in Japan.

Management of CKD requires multi-disciplinary involvement; therefore, we have done a strategic outcome study for CKD patients: Frontier of Renal Outcome Modifications in Japan study [21]. In this study, we prospectively observed the effects of intervention from dietitians and supportive care in CKD patients in addition to usual care recommended by Japanese Society of Nephrology and published practical guidebook with full involvement from the dietitian's society [22]. Furthermore, we joined the CKD outcomes and practice patterns (CKDopps) study to minimize the clinical complications in patients with advanced CKD and improving the transition to ESRD [23]. This study is being carried out in Brazil, France, Germany, and the United States. It aims to establish a multinational infrastructure for research, collaboration, and ancillary investigation.

Intervention Study

Asymptomatic hyperuricemia becomes one of the clinical topics as the new non-purine selective xanthine oxidase inhibitor. Hyperuricemia is well controlled even in advanced stages of CKD. Several studies reported the beneficial effect on CKD progression [24, 25]. However, we need more data to confirm it [26, 27], such as the final report of the FEATHER (FEbuxostat versus placebo rAndomized controlled Trial regarding reduced renal function in patients with Hyperuricemia complicated by CKD stage 3) study conducted in Japan [28]. According to the preliminary report, however, there were no significant differences in primary and secondary outcomes [29].

Also, other interesting studies evaluating the vascular function under uric acid control using the xanthine oxidase is ongoing [30]. Hyperuricemia may be viewed as a clinically important risk factor for various CVDs. The FREED (Febuxostat for Cerebral and Cardiorenovascular Events Prevention Study) study of 3 years duration, investigating an elderly Japanese population (febuxostat vs.

allopurinol), with a composite of CVD and renal events, and all deaths is currently under process [31].

Outcome Modifications in Japan study achieved behavior modification of CKD patients, namely, significantly lower discontinuous clinical visits, and behavior modification of both GPs and nephrologists, namely, significantly higher referral and co-treatment rates, resulting in the retardation of CKD progression, especially in patients with proteinuric Stage 3 CKD [32].

Conclusion

Hyperuricemia is a marker of unhealthy lifestyle, and subjects with hyperuricemia may develop CKD, ESRD, and CVD. However, the strength of hyperuricemia as a single risk factor is weaker than that of proteinuria and hypertension [1, 33]. Mechanisms of kidney damage by hyperuricemia are not certain yet. Both crystal- and non-crystal-dependent mechanism may be playing a role [34]. Larger and well-designed RCTs of UA-lowering therapy will be warranted to assess the precise renoprotective effects of the therapy [35].

References

1 Iseki K, Iseki C, Ikemiya Y, et al: Risk of developing end-stage renal disease in a cohort of mass screening. Kidney Int 1996;49:800–805.
2 Iseki K: The Okinawa screening program. J Am Soc Nephrol 2003;14(suppl 2):S127–S130.
3 Iseki K, Asahi K, Yamagata K, et al: Mortality Risk Among Screened Subjects of the Specific Health Check and Guidance Program in Japan 2008–2012. Clin Exp Nephrol 2017 (in press).
4 Iseki K, Iseki C, Kinjo K: Changes in serum uric acid have a reciprocal effect on eGFR change: a 10-year follow-up study of community-based screening in Okinawa, Japan. Hypertens Res 2013;36:650–654.
5 Kamei K, Konta T, Hirayama A, et al: A slight increase within the normal range of serum uric acid and the decline in renal function: associations in a community-based population. Nephrol Dial Transplant 2014;29:2286–2292.
6 Iseki K, Oshiro S, Tozawa M, et al: Significance of hyperuricemia on the early detection of renal failure in a cohort of screened subjects. Hypertens Res 2001;24:691–697.
7 Iseki K, Ikemiya Y, Inoue T, et al: Significance of hyperuricemia as a risk factor for developing ESRD in a screened cohort. Am J Kidney Dis 2004;44:642–650.
8 Nagahama K, Iseki K, Inoue T, et al: Hyperuricemia and cardiovascular risk factor clustering in a screened cohort in Okinawa, Japan. Hypertens Res 2004;27:227–234.
9 Nagahama K, Inoue T, Iseki K, et al: Hyperuricemia as a predictor of hypertension in a screened cohort in Okinawa, Japan. Hypertens Res 2004;27:835–841.
10 Nagahama K, Inoue T, Kohagura K, et al: Associations between serum uric acid levels and the incidence of hypertension and metabolic syndrome: a 4-year follow-up study of a large screened cohort in Okinawa, Japan. Hypertens Res 2015;38:213–218.

11 Nagahama K, Inoue T, Kohagura K, et al: Hyperuricemia predicts future metabolic syndrome: a 4-year follow-up study of a large screened cohort in Okinawa, Japan. Hypertens Res 2014;37:232–238.
12 Kohagura K, Kochi M, Miyagi T, et al: An association between uric acid levels and renal arteriolopathy in chronic kidney disease: a biopsy-based study. Hypertens Res 2013;36: 43–49.
13 Takae K, Nagata M, Hata J, et al: Serum uric acid as a risk factor for chronic kidney disease in a Japanese community. Circ J 2016;80: 1857–1862.
14 Kuriyama S, Maruyama Y, Nishio S, et al: Serum uric acid and the incidence of CKD and hypertension. Clin Exp Nephrol 2015;19: 1127–1234.
15 Li L, Chang A, Rostand SG, et al: A within-patient analysis for time-varying risk factors of CKD progression. J Am Soc Nephrol 2014; 25:606–613.
16 Krolewski AS: Progressive renal decline: the new paradigm of diabetic nephropathy in type 1 diabetes. Diabetes Care 2015;38:954–962.
17 Kamei K, Konta T, Hirayama A, et al: Associations between serum uric acid levels and the incidence of nonfatal stroke: a nationwide community-based cohort study. Clin Exp Nephrol 2016;21:497–503.
18 Kamei K, Konta T, Ichikawa K, et al: Serum uric acid levels and mortality in the Japanese population: the Yamagata (Takahata) study. Clin Exp Nephrol 2016;20:904–909.
19 Kawasoe S, Kubozono T, Yoshifuku S, et al: Uric acid level and prevalence of atrial fibrillation in a Japanese general population of 285,882. Circ J 2016;80:2453–2459.
20 Hara S, Tsuji H, Ohmoto Y, et al: High serum uric acid level and low urine pH as predictors of metabolic syndrome: a retrospective cohort study in a Japanese urban population. Metabolism 2012;61:281–288.
21 Yamagata K, Makino H, Akizawa T, et al: Design and methods of a strategic outcome study for chronic kidney disease: frontier of renal outcome modifications in Japan. Clin Exp Nephrol 2014;14:144–151.
22 Iseki K, Yamagata K: A practical guide of salt and protein restriction for CKD patients in Japan. BMC Nephrol 2016;17:87
23 Mariani L, Stengel B, Combe C, et al: The CKD outcomes and practice patterns study (CKDopps): rationale and methods. Am J Kidney Dis 2016;68:402–413.
24 Tanaka K, Nakayama M, Kanno M, et al: Renoprotective effects of febuxostat in hyperuricemic patients with chronic kidney disease: a parallel-group, randomized, controlled trial. Clin Exp Nephrol 2015;19: 1044–1053.
25 Sircar D, Chatterjee S, Waikhom R, et al: Efficacy of febuxostat for slowing the GFR decline in patients with CKD and asymptomatic hyperuricemia: a 6-month, double-blind, randomized, placebo-controlled trial. Am J Kidney Dis 2015;66:945–650.
26 Badve SV, Brown F, Hawley CM, et al: Challenges of conducting a trial of uric-acid-lowering therapy in CKD. Nat Rev Nephrol 2011; 7:295–300.
27 Bose B, Badve SV, Hiremath SS, et al: Effects of uric acid-lowering therapy on renal outcomes: a systematic review and meta-analysis. Nephrol Dial Transplant 2014;29:406–413.
28 Hosoya T, Kimura K, Itoh S, et al: The effect of febuxostat to prevent a further reduction in renal function of patients with hyperuricemia who have never had gout and are complicated by chronic kidney disease stage 3: study protocol for a multicenter randomized controlled study. Trials 2014;15:26–34.
29 Hosoya T, Kimura K: Effect of febuxostat on the progression of GFR in CKD patients associated with hyperuricemia: randomized double blind placebo controlled study. Jpn J Nephrol 2017;59:267.
30 Hosoya T, Oyama J, Tanaka A, Sato Y, et al: Rationale and design of a multicenter randomized study for evaluating vascular function under uric acid control using the xanthine oxidase inhibitor, febuxostat: the PRIZE study. Cardiovasc Diabetol 2016;15: 87–96.
31 Kojima S, Matsui K, Ogawa H, et al: Rationale, design, and baseline characteristics of a study to evaluate the effect of febuxostat in preventing cerebral, cardiovascular, and renal events in patients with hyperuricemia. J Cardiol 2017;69:169–175.

32 Yamagata K, Makino H, Iseki K, et al: Effect of behavior modification on outcome in early- to moderate-stage chronic hidney disease: a cluster-randomized trial. PLoS One 2016; 11:e0151422.
33 Tozawa M, Iseki K, Iseki C, et al: Blood pressure predicts risk of developing end-stage renal disease in men and women. Hypertension 2003;41:1341–1345.
34 Hisatome I, Kuwabara M: Hyperuricemia plays pivotal role in progression of kidney disease. Circ J 2016;80:1710–1711.
35 Kumagai T, Ota T, Tamura Y, et al: Time to target uric acid to retard CKD progression. Clin Exp Nephrol 2017;21:182–192.

Kunitoshi Iseki
Clinical Research Support Center, Tomishiro Central Hospital
25 Ueta, Tomigusuku
Okinawa 901–0243 (Japan)
E-Mail chihokun_ohra@yahoo.co.jp

Treviño-Becerra A, Iseki K (eds): Uric Acid in Chronic Kidney Disease.
Contrib Nephrol. Basel, Karger, 2018, vol 192, pp 48–55 (DOI: 10.1159/000484278)

Hyperuricemia and Progression of Chronic Kidney Disease: Role of Phenotype Transition of Renal Tubular and Endothelial Cells

Duk-Hee Kang

Division of Nephrology, Department of Internal Medicine, Ewha Woman's University College of Medicine, Ewha Medical Research Center, Seoul, Korea

Abstract

Background: Although the clinical implication of hyperuricemia in chronic kidney disease has been an issue of active debate, recent data suggested a causative role of uric acid (UA) in the development of renal disease. Afferent arteriopathy, an induction of oxidative stress and an activation of local inflammation, have been regarded as the mechanisms of UA-induced renal disease, which contribute to glomerular hypertrophy and interstitial fibrosis via endothelial dysfunction. However, there have been rare studies on the direct effect of UA on phenotype transition of renal cells such as epithelial-to-mesenchymal transition (EMT) or endothelial-to-mesenchymal transition (EndoMT). ***Summary:*** We have reported that UA-induced EMT of cultured renal tubular cells, which was blocked by the organic anion transport inhibitor, probenecid. UA increased the expression of snail and slug, the transcriptional repressors of E-cadherin, which resulted in a downregulation of E-cadherin production. UA also increased the degradation of E-cadherin via ubiquitination. UA also induced EndoMT with an increase in ROS generation and glycocalyx shedding of cultured vascular endothelial cells. Treatment with antioxidants ameliorated UA-induced EndoMT. In the kidney of hyperuricemic rats, there was an evidence of EMT before the development of significant tubulointerstitial fibrosis, as shown by decreased E-cadherin expression and an increased α-smooth muscle actin (α-SMA) in renal tubular cells. Allopurinol significantly inhibited UA-induced EMT with an amelioration of renal fibrosis. In addition, endothelial staining in peritubular capillaries (PTC) was substantially decreased with de-novo expression of α-SMA in endothelial cells of PTC. ***Key Messages:*** UA per se induced a phenotypic transition of epithelial and endothelial cells via an induction of oxidative stress and glycocalyx shedding, which could be one of the mechanisms of UA-induced kidney disease.

Introduction

The prevalence of hyperuricemia (HU) has substantially increased during the recent 20 years, and it has become one of the emerging clinical concerns in the world [1]. Uric acid (UA)-related researches including basic, epidemiologic and clinical studies to understand the role of UA in the development of cardiovascular, renal and metabolic diseases flourished during the last decades [2–6]. Despite the different strength of evidence in each individual studies, epidemiologic studies repeatedly and consistently show HU to be an independent risk factor for hypertension and kidney disease [7, 8]. And, longitudinal studies demonstrate UA as a risk factor for the onset and progression of kidney disease (reviewed in [9]). However, since a decreased glomerular filtration rate is one the strongest among the risk factors predicting HU, the clinical implication of elevated UA levels in patients with chronic kidney disease (CKD) has been an issue of active debate. Although substantial progress has been made on our understandings on UA, we still do have many questions unanswered at this moment, which include the mechanism of UA-induced kidney disease. Previous investigations have suggested that HU may induce renal injury by causing endothelial dysfunction, an induction of oxidative stress and local inflammation [4, 10]. Further studies also demonstrated afferent arteriolar thickening and hyalinosis of the preglomerular arterioles of the kidney, often accompanied by glomerular hypertrophy via an activation of renin-angiotensin system [11]. A decreased production of nitric oxide and impaired vasodilatation also lead to an impaired renal blood flow, renal ischemia, and ultimately renal fibrosis. In addition to this hemodynamic alteration as an indirect mechanism of UA-induced renal disease, the direct effect of UA on residential cells in the kidney, especially phenotype transition of each cell such as epithelial-to-mesenchymal transition (EMT) and endothelial-to-mesenchymal transition (EndoMT), could play a role in the development of renal injury in HU.

UA-Induced EMT of Renal Tubular Cells

Many factors mediating renal fibrosis such as high glucose, hypoxia, profibrotic cytokines, and inflammatory mediators have direct effects on renal tubules. Some profibrogenic factors induce phenotypic transition of renal tubules, which is known as EMT [12]. EMT is one of the earliest phenomena of renal fibrosis observed before the development of significant changes in renal pathology, and has been considered a therapeutic target due to its reversible characteristic [12,

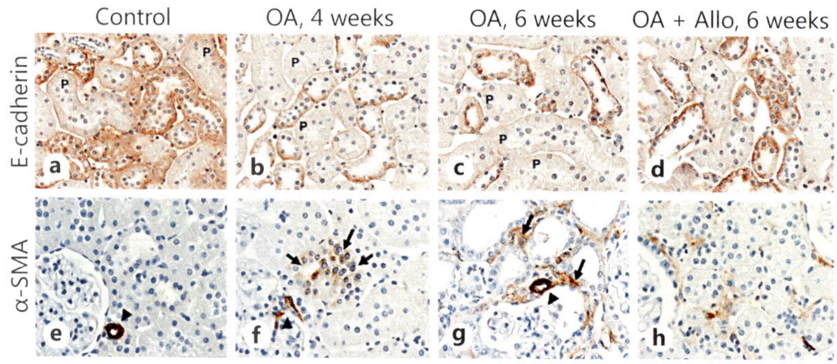

Fig. 1. UA-induced EMT in hyperuricemic rats. Representative immunohistochemistry of E-cadherin (**a–d**) and α-SMA (**e–h**) staining in control rats (**a**, **e**) and rats in 4 weeks (**b**, **f**) and 6 weeks (**c**, **g**) of OA feeding. E-cadherin staining in renal tubules was decreased in proximal tubules (P) and other cortical tubules with de novo expression of α-SMA in the cytoplasm of some renal tubules (**f**, arrows) and interstitial area (**g**, arrows). The normal expression of α-SMA in VSMC of arteriole is shown (arrowheads). Allopurinol treatment ameliorated an altered expression of E-cadherin (**d**) and α-SMA (**h**) in hyperuricemic rats (6 weeks; modified from reference [16]). UA, uric acid; EMT, epithelial-to-mesenchymal transition; OA, oxonic acid; α-SMA, α-smooth muscle actin.

13]. EMT is generally characterized by a decrease in the expressions of epithelial markers such as E-cadherin and zonula occludens protein with de novo acquisition of α-smooth muscle actin (α-SMA) [14, 15].

We found the phenotypic transition of renal tubules before the development of renal dysfunction and significant tubulointerstitial fibrosis in hyperuricemic rats fed on uricase inhibitor, oxonic acid (OA), which was ameliorated by the UA-lowering therapy [16]. In 4 weeks of OA treatment, the expression of α-SMA and vimentin was observed in the cytoplasm of some renal tubules along with a decrease in E-cadherin expression. In 6 weeks of OA administration, the evidence of EMT of renal tubules became evident with the development of interstitial fibrosis, an elevation of BUN and creatinine in HU rats, which was alleviated by xanthine oxidase inhibitor, allopurinol (Fig. 1). In cultured renal tubular cells (NRK cells), a loss of cell adhesion was the first finding observed as early as 24 h of UA exposure, followed by morphologic change into elongated fibroblastoid cells. Phenotypic transition of NRK cells was associated with the de novo expression of α-SMA as well as a significant decrease in E-cadherin [16]. Importantly, pretreatment with probenecid (which blocked the entry of UA into cells) significantly inhibited the UA-induced changes in the expression of E-cadherin and α-SMA in NRK cells, suggesting that UA per se entering into cells was responsible for UA-induced EMT. UA not only inhibited the transcription of E-cadherin mRNA via an induction of Snail and Slug but also enhanced the degradation of E-cadherin [16]. During EMT, an initial decrease in E-cadherin levels likely occurs by lysosomal degradation [17–19]. Lysosomal degradation was known to be associated with ubiquitination of E-cadherin [19], which was also found in UA-stimulated NRK cells. We have demonstrated UA-induced downregulation of E-cadherin mRNA as early as 6 hours, followed by E-cadherin ubiquitination and degradation at 24 and 48 h respectively.

UA-Induced EndoMT of Endothelial Cells of Peritubular Capillaries

More recent studies have suggested the phenotype transition of endothelial cells as an emerging mechanism of vascular and renal disease via EndoMT [20]. Endothelial lineage tracing further demonstrated that EndoMT was an important mechanism contributing to the accumulation of activated fibroblasts and myofibroblasts in kidney fibrosis. Several studies have verified the presence of EndoMT in various animal models of renal fibrosis including diabetic nephropathy and unilateral ureteral obstruction [21, 22]; however, it has not been investigated whether UA induced EndoMT.

Our data showed that UA induced the changes in cell morphology of human umbilical vein endothelial cells (HUVEC) from a typical cobblestone shape to elongated spindle-shaped cells with a loss of cell-to-cell contact (Fig. 2). In association with morphologic transition, UA decreased the mRNA and protein expression of VE-cadherin with an induction of de novo expression of α-SMA (Fig. 2). Pretreatment with probenecid blocked the UA-induced EndoMT. A key mechanism of UA-induced EndoMT seems to be an induction of oxidative stress. Antioxidants such as NAC, apocynin, and mitotempo ameliorated UA-induced EndoMT. Interestingly, UA increased glycocalyx shedding of HUVEC from 6 h shown as a decreased staining of lectin. Glycocalyx is a fuzzy coat-like covering extending approximately 50–100 nm into the lumen of a blood vessel, which is connected to the endothelium through proteoglycans and glycoproteins and it plays the first-line defense against endothelial injury [23]. Glycocalyx is an important determinant of vascular permeability; it also contributes to maintain healthy vascular endothelium by the inhibition of thrombosis, reducing ROS generation and maintaining the bioavailability of nitric oxide.

In the animal model of HU, there was a decrease in endothelial RECA staining in peritubular capillaries (PTC). At the same time, some endothelial cells in PTC showed de novo staining of α-SMA, the markers of mesenchymal cells, sug-

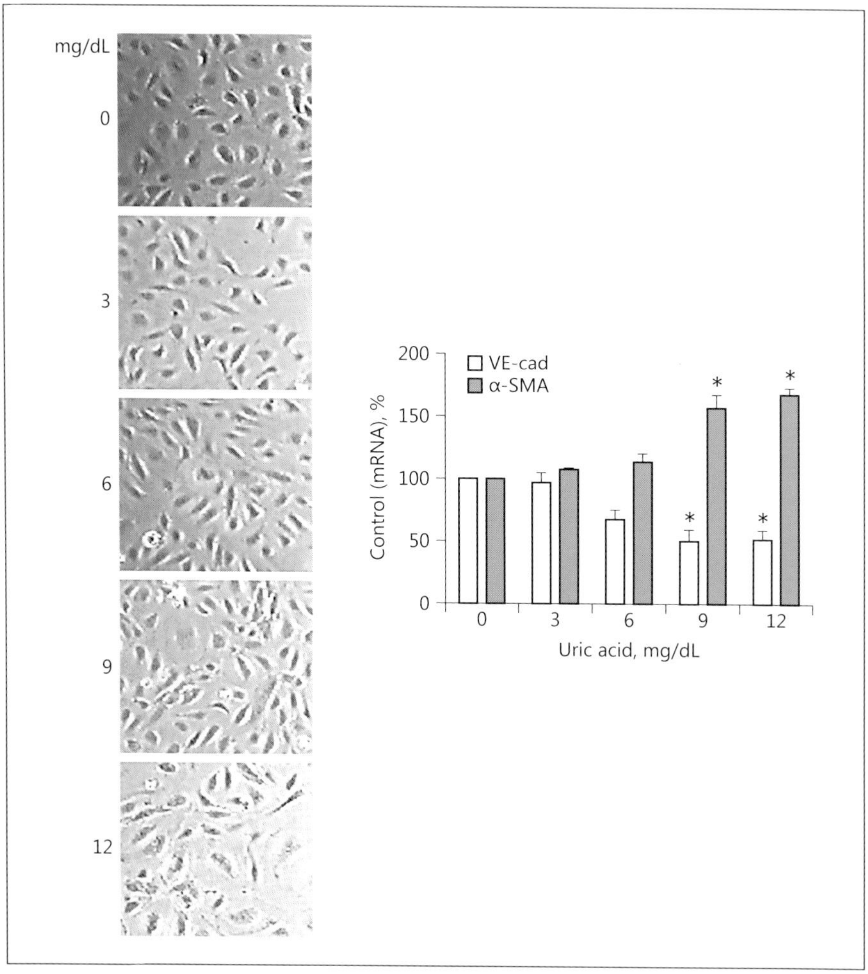

Fig. 2. UA-induced EndoMT and Glycocalyx Shedding in HUVECs. UA (>9 mg/dL) induces a phenotypic transition of HUVEC to elongated fibroblast-like cells from cuboidal cobble stone-shaped cells at 48 h. UA induces the changes in mRNA expression of VE-cadherin and α-SMA from 24 h (*n* = 5). UA, uric acid; HUVEC, human umbilical vein endothelial cell; α-SMA, α-smooth muscle actin.

gesting the presence of EndoMT in the kidney of hyperuricemic rats. Allopurinol treatment partially reversed EndoMT in hyperuricemic rats.

We have also shown that UA per se induced the senescence and apoptosis of HUVEC via an activation of local activation of renin-angiotensin system and oxidative stress [24]. These findings suggest the direct effect of UA on vascular endothelial cells to induce oxidative stress, ROS generation, and glycocalyx shedding, which lead to EndoMT, cell aging, and ultimately cell death.

Other Types of Phenotype Transitions in HU

We have previously reported that UA increased proliferation of vascular smooth muscle cells with an induction of inflammatory phenotype shown as an increased MCP-1 and COX-2 and de novo expression of C-reactive protein [2, 10, 25]. Increased ED-1 positive macrophages were also observed in VSMCs in hyperuricemic rats. Original phenotype of VSMC should be contractile but switched into synthetic and inflammatory phenotype upon UA exposure.

Not closely related to the progression of CKD, we have already published the phenotype transition of hepatocyte to accumulate triglyceride with an induction of key enzymes of fatty acid synthesis by UA. An induction of endoplasmic reticulum stress and oxidative stress in hepatocytes by UA was found to contribute to UA-induced non-alcoholic fatty liver disease [26]. Adipocytes also showed an evidence of phenotype transition. UA accelerated the maturation of preadipocytes with a decrease in adiponectin expression, which led to the acquisition of diabetic phenotype [27].

Conclusion

UA imposed the direct effects on various residential cells in the kidney. EMT of renal tubular cells by UA could also be a mechanism of an accumulation of mesenchymal cells, which accelerated the production of extracellular matrix and renal fibrosis. UA-induced EndoMT also potentially contribute to the development of renal ischemia via an impaired vasodilatation and rarefaction of PTC, which result in the development of fibrosis.

Further studies to verify whether immunohistochemistric evidences of EMT, EndoMT, and other forms of phenotype transition contribute to the development of renal disease in HU will be needed.

Acknowledgment

This work was supported by a grant received from National Research Foundation of Korea (NRF) grant funded by the Korea government (MSIP; NRF-2015R1A2A1A15053374, NRF-2017R1A2B2005849).

Disclosure Statement

The authors have no conflicts of interest to declare.

References

1 Zhu Y, Pandya BJ, Choi HK: Prevalence of gout and hyperuricemia in the US general population: the National Health and Nutrition Examination Survey 2007–2008. Arthritis Rheum 2011;63:3136–3141.

2 Kang DH, Nakagawa T, Feng L, Watanabe S, Han L, Mazzali M, Truong L, Harris R, Johnson RJ: A role for uric acid in the progression of renal disease. J Am Soc Nephrol 2002;3: 2888–2897.

3 Goicoechea M, de Vinuesa SG, Verdalles U, Ruiz-Caro C, Ampuero J, Rincon A, Arroyo D, Luno J: Effect of allopurinol in chronic kidney disease progression and cardiovascular risk. Clin J Am Soc Nephrol 2010;5:1388–1393.

4 Feig D, Kang DH, Johnson RJ: Uric acid and cardiovascular risk. N Engl J Med 2008;59: 1811–1821.

5 Iseki K, Ikemiya Y, Inoue T, Iseki C, Kinjo K, Takishita S: Significance of hyperuricemia as a risk factor for developing ESRD in a screened cohort. Am J Kidney Dis 2004;44: 642–650.

6 Kanbay M, Jensen T, Solak Y, Le M, Roncal-Jimenez C, Rivard C, Lanaspa MA, Nakagawa T, Johnson RJ: Uric acid in metabolic syndrome: From an innocent bystander to a central player. Eur J Intern Med 2016;29:3–8.

7 Grayson PC, Kim SY, LaValley M, Choi HK: Hyperuricemia and incident hypertension: a systematic review and meta-analysis. Arthritis Care Res (Hoboken). 2011;63:102–110.

8 Johnson RJ, Nakagawa T, Jalal D, Sánchez-Lozada LG, Kang DH, Ritz E: Uric acid and chronic kidney disease: which is chasing which? Nephrol Dial Transplant 2013;28: 2221–2228.

9 Kanji T, Gandhi M, Clase CM, Yang R: Urate lowering therapy to improve renal outcomes in patients with chronic kidney disease: systematic review and meta-analysis. BMC Nephrol 2015;16:58–67.

10 Kang DH, Park SK, Lee IK, Johnson R: Uric acid-induced C-reactive protein: Implication on cell proliferation and nitric oxide production of human vascular cells. J Am Soc Nephrol 2005;16:3553–3562.

11 Mazzali M, Kanellis J, Han L, Feng L, Xia YY, Chen Q, Kang DH, Gordon KL, Watanabe S, Nakagawa T, Lan HY, Johnson RJ: Hyperuricemia induces a primary arteriolopathy in rats by a blood pressure-independent mechanism. Am J Physiol Renal Physiol 2002; 282:F991–F997.

12 Liu Y: Epithelial to mesenchymal transition in renal fibrogenesis: pathologic significance, molecular mechanism, and therapeutic intervention. J Am Soc Nephrol 2004;15:1–12.

13 Liu Y: New insights into epithelial-mesenchymal transition in kidney fibrosis. J Am Soc Nephrol 2010;21:212–222.

14 Zeisberg M, Duffield JS: Resolved: EMT produces fibroblasts in the kidney. J Am Soc Nephrol 2010;21:1247–1253.

15 Zeisberg M, Kalluri R: The role of epithelial-to-mesenchymal transition in renal fibrosis. J Mol Med 2004;82:175–181.

16 Yu ES, Kim MJ, Shin HS, Jang YH, Choi HS, Jo I, Johnson RJ, Kang DH: Uric acid-induced phenotypic transition of renal tubular cells as a novel mechanism of chronic kidney disease. Am J Physiol Renal Physiol 2013; 304:F471–F480.

17 Palacios F, Tushir JS, Fujita Y, D'Souza-Schorey C: Lysosomal targeting of E-cadherin: a unique mechanism for the down-regulation of cell-cell adhesion during epithelial to mesenchymal transitions. Mol Cell Biol 2005;25: 389–402.

18 Janda E, Nevolo M, Lehmann K, Downward J, Beug H, Grieco M: Raf plus TGFβ-dependent EMT is initiated by endocytosis and lysosomal degradation of E-cadherin. Oncogene 2006;25:7117–7130.

19 Shen Y, Hirsch DS, Sasiela CA, Wu WJ: Cdc42 regulates E-cadherin ubiquitination and degradation through an epidermal growth factor receptor to Src-mediated pathway. J Biol Chem 2008;283:5127–5137.

20 Zeisberg EM, Potenta SE, Sugimoto H, Zeisberg M, Kalluri R: Fibroblasts in kidney fibrosis emerge via endothelial-to-mesenchymal transition. J Am Soc Nephrol 2008;19: 2282–2287.

21 Li J, Qu X, Bertram JF: Endothelial-myofibroblast transition contributes to the early development of diabetic renal interstitial fibrosis in streptozotocin-induced diabetic mice. Am J Pathol 2009;175:1380–1388.

22 O'Riordan E, Mendelev N, Patschan S, Patschan D, Eskander J, Cohen-Gould L, Chander P, Goligorsky MS: Chronic NOS inhibition actuates endothelial-mesenchymal transformation. Am J Physiol Heart Circ Physiol 2007;292:H285–H294.
23 Tarbell JM, Cancel LM: The glycocalyx and its significance in human medicine. J Intern Med 2016;280:97–113.
24 Yu MA, Sánchez-Lozada LG, Johnson RJ, Kang DH: Oxidative stress with an activation of the renin-angiotensin system in human vascular endothelial cells as a novel mechanism of uric acid-induced endothelial dysfunction. J Hypertens 2010;28:1234–1242.
25 Kanellis J, Watanabe S, Li JH, Kang DH, Li P, Nakagawa T, Wamsley A, Sheikh-Hamad D, Lan HY, Feng L, Johnson RJ: Uric acid stimulates monocyte chemoattractant protein-1 production in vascular smooth muscle cells via mitogen-activated protein kinase and cyclooxygenase-2. Hypertension 2003;41:1287–1293.
26 Choi YJ, Shin HS, Choi HS, Park JW, Jo I, Oh ES, Lee KY, Lee BH, Johnson RJ, Kang DH: Uric acid induces fat accumulation via generation of endoplasmic reticulum stress and SREBP-1c activation in hepatocytes. Lab Invest 2014;94:1114–1125.
27 Sautin YY, Nakagawa T, Zharikov S, Johnson RJ: Adverse effects of the classic antioxidant uric acid in adipocytes: NADPH oxidase-mediated oxidative/nitrosative stress. Am J Physiol Cell Physiol 2007;293:C584–C596.

Duk-Hee Kang, MD, PhD
Division of Nephrology, Ewha University College of Medicine
911 Mok-dong Yangcheon-Ku
Seoul 158-710 (Korea)
E-Mail dhkang@ewha.ac.kr

Treviño-Becerra A, Iseki K (eds): Uric Acid in Chronic Kidney Disease.
Contrib Nephrol. Basel, Karger, 2018, vol 192, pp 56–68 (DOI: 10.1159/000484279)

Time to Target Uric Acid to Retard Chronic Kidney Disease Progression

Shunya Uchida[a] · Takanori Kumagai[a, b] · Wen Xiu Chang[c] · Yoshifuru Tamura[a] · Shigeru Shibata[a]

[a]Department of Internal Medicine, Teikyo University School of Medicine, Tokyo, [b]Support for Community Medicine Endowed Chair, Teikyo University School of Medicine, Tokyo, and [c]Department of Nephrology, Tianjin First Center Hospital, Tianjin, China

Abstract

Uric acid (UA) remains a risk factor for the progression of chronic kidney disease (CKD). Most observational studies showed a slight elevation in the serum UA level and this independently predicts the incidence and development of CKD. The recent meta-analysis, however, did not reach the conclusion that urate-lowering therapy with allopurinol retards the progression of CKD. The target level of serum UA if treated is another issue of debate. Our recent analysis by propensity score analysis has shown that the serum UA should be targeted below 6.0 mg/dL to inhibit the progression towards end-stage renal disease. Underlying mechanisms whereby an increase in serum UA induces kidney injury have been elucidated in animal models. Hyperuricemic models can lead to systemic hypertension, arteriolosclerosis including afferent arteriolopathy as well as albuminuria probably due to the activation of oxidative stress. Discoveries of urate transporters have elucidated the novel mechanism of UA transport in the kidney and intestine. The intestinal ABCG2 may play a compensatory role in light of decreased renal clearance of UA in CKD model rats, the trigger of which is not a uremic toxin but serum UA itself. Insulin directly upregulates URAT1 and downregulates ABCG2 in the kidney tubules, suggesting a possible link between UA and metabolic syndrome. This review summarizes the recent knowledge on the causal effect of serum UA on the kidney injury.

Introduction

Chronic kidney disease (CKD) is a major public health problem worldwide and the prevalence of CKD in the general population ranges from 8 to 16%. The unfavorable impact of CKD includes not only progression to end-stage renal disease (ESRD) but also increased risk of cardiovascular disease. Early recognition and intervention against risk factors involved in the progression of CKD are crucial to improve renal outcomes of patients at risk. A line of evidence has shown major risk factors for subsequent incidence of ESRD such as anemia, proteinuria, and hypertension in addition to precedent kidney dysfunction [1]. However, the second-line risk predictors remain to be elucidated with candidates being hypoalbuminemia, hyperphosphatemia, metabolic acidosis, dyslipidemia, diabetes, and hyperuricemia as well.

Recently, the relationship between hyperuricemia and CKD has attracted much attention amid ever-increasing experimental and clinical data. The debate, however, continues regarding whether hyperuricemia plays a causal role in the progression of CKD or is simply a marker of renal dysfunction [2]. In this review, we will describe the up-to-date knowledge on the impact of uric acid (UA) on the progression of CKD both in basic and clinical experiments and demonstrate a line of evidence when and how to target serum UA (SUA) in order to inhibit the progression of CKD.

Pathophysiology of Hyperuricemia in CKD

Hyperuricemia has been conceptually classified into 2 types; overproduction and underexcretion. In general, approximately two-thirds of UA is excreted through the kidneys and the remaining one-third is discharged through the intestinal tract, whereas excretion from the bile duct accounts for less than 5% of all excretion. However, the kinetics of UA in decreased renal excretion in CKD remains to be elucidated. We recently demonstrated that ABCG2 mRNA expression in the intestine increases in 5/6 nephrectomized rats, suggesting the compensatory increased elimination of UA from the intestine in the context of decreased renal clearance of UA, so that SUA level in the CKD rats is kept constant as the control [3, 4]. Moreover, the trigger to induce intestinal ABCG2 mRNA was assumed to be SUA itself but not a kind of uremic toxin because hyperuricemic model rats made by oxonic acid loading stimulated ABCG2 mRNA to a greater degree than that of 5/6 nephrectomized rats [4]. In those experiments URAT1, GLUT9, ABCG2, and NPT4 in the proximal tubules uniformly decreased in the expression of both mRNA and immunohistochemistry probably due to the CKD-associated tubular injury [4]. The result indicates that tubular urate transporters do not play a principal role in causing CKD-induced hyperuricemia, which simply results from the decrease in glomerular filtrated UA [3].

Hyperuricemia is well known to associate with metabolic syndrome whose underlying derangement is considered insulin resistance or hyperinsulinemia.

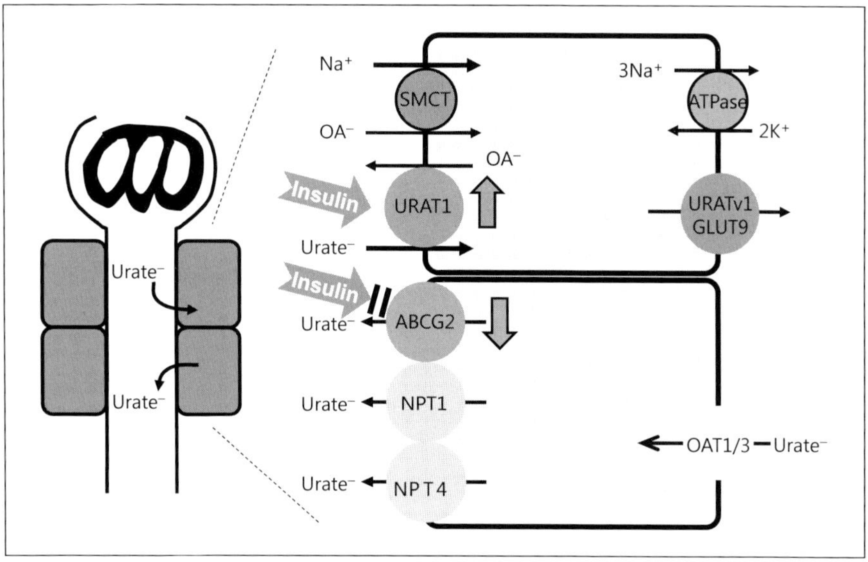

Fig. 1. Insulin directly stimulates URAT1 and inhibits ABCG2 urate transporters. Renal proximal tubules transport glomerular-filtrated urate through specific urate transporters. Urate is reabsorbed by URAT1 at the luminal membrane and is expelled by GLUT9 (a.k.a. URATv1) at the basolateral membrane. Meanwhile, intracellular urate is secreted by several urate exporters such as ABCG2, NPT1 and NPT4. Subcutaneous infusion of insulin directly upregulates URAT1 and downregulates ABCG2, both leading to increase in serum uric acid. Other urate transporters play a marginal role in insulin administration. This scheme is consistent with the fact that high incidence of hyperuricemia is linked to metabolic syndrome whose underlying pathophysiology is insulin resistance or hyperinsulinemia.

A line of evidence suggests that a novel antidiabetic drug, sodium-glucose transporter 2 (SGLT2) inhibitor shows certain decline in SUA. The mechanism by which SGLT2 inhibitor causes decline in SUA is attributed to uricosuria due to glycosuria, but the detailed mechanism remains largely unknown. One possibility is the inhibition of urate reabsorption via GLUT9 isoform located at the luminal membrane of the proximal tubule in the background of a high glucose microenvironment [5]. Using the animal model, we attempted to investigate the mechanism by which SGLT2 inhibitor, ipragliflozin, decreases the SUA level in association with the altered regulation of urate transporters in the kidney. At first, streptozotocin-induced diabetic model rats were utilized. Given the extremely lowered level of SUA in the rats, SUA level itself did not decrease further, but we could see the significant changes in the expression of urate transporters, decrease in URAT1 and increase in ABCG2, in response to insulin treatment [6] as shown in Figure 1. The finding is not contradictory to the fact that hyperuricemia is associated with metabolic syndrome such as obesity, diabetes, hyperlipidemia, and hypertension [7, 8]. Given the possible increase in SUA level by hyperinsulinemia, the selection of the diabetic drugs will be the further consideration of drug choice in the diabetic patients. It is conjectured that possible drugs to increase the insulin level includes sulfonyl urea in addition to insulin.

Mechanisms by Which Hyperuricemia Causes the Progression of CKD in Basic Research

Basic research suggested that hyperuricemia induces renal injury through multiple crystal-independent mechanisms involving renal vasoconstriction mediated by endothelial dysfunction, activation of the renin-angiotensin system, afferent arteriolopathy, and epithelial-to-mesenchymal transition in renal tubular cells.

The molecule of UA, which may act as a strong antioxidant in the extracellular environment, may be a pro-oxidant inside the cell where it can stimulate NADPH oxidases [9, 10]. Oxidative stress induced by hyperuricemia decreases endothelial nitric oxide (eNO) bioactivity leading to endothelial dysfunction [9]. Animal models by administering oxonic acid revealed that hyperuricemia increases cyclooxygenase 2 expression, leading to the proliferation of vascular smooth muscle cells in preglomerular arteries [11]. In addition, hyperuricemia increases renin activity, leading to the upregulation of angiotensin II, which also causes the proliferation of vascular smooth muscle cells [11, 12]. Preglomerular vasculopathy by hyperuricemia deranges the autoregulatory response of afferent arterioles, leading to glomerular hypertension [9, 13, 14]. Vascular wall thickening by hyperuricemia also leads to lumen obliteration and hypoperfusion of the kidney, resulting in tubulointerstitial inflammation and fibrosis as well as arterial hypertension [14, 15]. UA can also induce epithelial-to-mesenchymal transition in renal tubular cells, leading to tubulointerstitial fibrosis [16]. In diabetic (db/db) mice that developed hyperuricemia, allopurinol reduced albuminuria and decreased tubulointerstitial injury [17], which is mediated by a reduction in inflammatory cells due to the reduction in intercellular adhesion molecule 1 expression by tubular epithelial cells [17]. The two sides of a coin of the role of UA are shown in Figure 2.

Of recent interest is the role of xanthine oxidase (XO) activity on cardiorenal protection independently of SUA because XO directly influences oxidative stress by generating superoxide free radicals as one of the reactive oxidative species. Several decades ago, Diamond et al. [18] demonstrated that allopurinol, XO

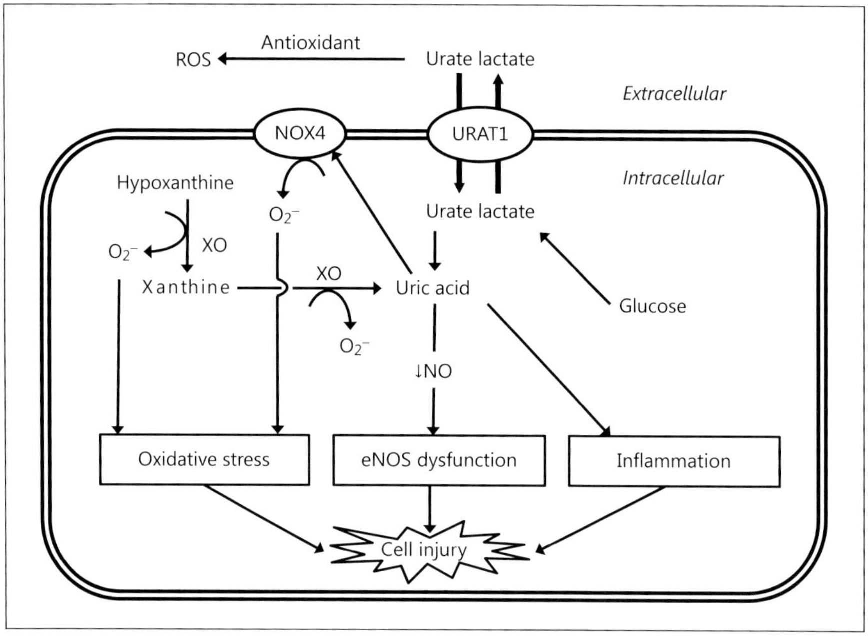

Fig. 2. Uric acid is antioxidant outside the cell and prooxidant within the cell. Uric acid is generated via xanthine oxidoreductase in the cell, inevitably yielding superoxide free radicals. Intracellular uric acid directly upregulates NOX4, resulting in the superoxide free radical as a distinct pathway. The oxidative stress causes cell injury, while uric acid decreases endothelial nitric oxide (NO) generation, leading to endothelial dysfunction.

inhibitor, dramatically decreased the proteinuria by 80% and ameliorated glomerular pathological abnormalities such as podocyte blebbing, segmental mesangial cell proliferation, and matrix expansion induced by puromycin aminonucleoside (PA).

We have recently reported that topiroxostat, a novel XO inhibitor, ameliorated proteinuria in association with podocyte injury markers such as decrease in WT-1 and podocin expressions and foot process effacement on electron microscope [19]. We further attempted to explore the role of oxidative stress in this particular setting. In association with PA treatment, several oxidative stress markers altered with increases in 8OHdG, nitrotyrosine, and NOX4 expressions in the kidney cortex. 8OHdG was increased in the glomerular epithelial cells and mesangial cells. The expression of XO also increased probably due to PA administration. Topiroxostat significantly decreased proteinuria level by a half and almost completely restored oxidative stress markers. Interestingly, UA level in the kidney cortex was doubly increased, suggesting that intracellular UA may be responsible for inducing the oxidative stress in the kidney cells including podocytes. Thus, podocytes in culture were stimulated by 12 mg/dL UA in the culture medium, causing NOX4 expression in the cells [19]. Taken altogether, the intracellular UA accumulation via activation of XO by PA injection triggers the generation of superoxide free radicals, while cellular UA activates NOX4 in the membrane, resulting in superoxide free radical generation through this independent pathway. This oxidative stress was almost all rescued by the administration of topiroxostat, resulting in the alleviation of massive proteinuria [19]. We believe that the elucidation of improvement of the disease progression of CKD by topiroxostat warrants further investigation in humans.

Relationship between Hyperuricemia and CKD in Observational Studies

The level of SUA increases as CKD progresses, but whether hyperuricemia plays a causal role in CKD progression remains to be elucidated [2, 20, 21]. Many large epidemiological studies have evaluated the association between SUA and the development or the progression of CKD (Table 1). Most observational studies showed positive results in which hyperuricemia is an independent risk factor for the development and progression of renal disease in patients with diabetes or without diabetes. A meta-analysis of 13 observational studies including 190,718 patients showed that hyperuricemia was an independent risk factor for the development of newly diagnosed CKD in non-CKD patients [22]. This association was stronger in Western countries than that in Asian populations [22]. This difference may be attributed to race, and geographical or diet differences, as the Western diet might contain more purine-rich foods. Interestingly, the subgroup of follow-up year revealed that the longer time period for observation, the greater the risk of the development of new-onset CKD in hyperuricemic patients, suggesting that hyperuricemia may accelerate CKD progression in the long-term perspective [22]. A cross-sectional study enrolling 3,212 T2DM patients showed that the prevalence of diabetic kidney disease was higher in hyperuricemic patients than in patients with normouricemia (68.3 vs. 41.5%) and increased with increasing SUA levels [23]. In addition, a GLUT9 polymorphism, which is strongly associated with SUA levels in healthy individuals of the general population with normal renal function strongly predicted the progression of CKD in a cohort of 755 patients with CKD [24]. This finding is compatible with the hypothesis that the link between hyperuricemia and CKD progression is causal in nature.

However, there are some observational studies that showed no significant relationship between hyperuricemia and progression of CKD [25]. A prospective analysis of the Mild to Moderate Kidney Disease study enrolling 177 patients with non-diabetic CKD revealed that hyperuricemia predicts CKD pro-

Table 1. Observational studies of hyperuricemia and CKD (cited from ref [25])

Author (year)	Participants (mean age, years)	Country; at risk	Design (follow-up, years)	Finding on SUA and kidney function	Statistical significance
Iseki (2001)	6,403 (48.3)	Japan; healthy	Retrospective cohort (2)	SUA >8 mg/dL increased CKD risk 3-fold in men and 10-fold in women	Yes
Iseki (2004)	48,177 (52.2)	Japan; healthy	Prospective cohort (6.75)	SUA >6 mg/dL was an independent predictor of ESRD in women (HR 5.770)	Yes
Domrongkitchaipron (2005)	3,499 (43.0)	Thailand; healthy	Prospective cohort (12)	SUA >6.3 mg/dL associated with 1.69-fold risk of progressive decline in renal function	Yes
Chonchol (2007)	5,808 (73)	USA; healthy	Prospective cohort (median 6.9)	SUA was strongly associated with prevalence but weakly with incidence of CKD	Yes
Obermayr (2008)	21,457 (42.5)	Austria; healthy	Prospective cohort (median 7)	SUA >7 mg/dL increased CKD risk 1.74-fold in men and 3.12-fold in women	Yes
Sturm (2008)	227 (46.4)	Europe; CKD 1,2,3,4	Prospective cohort (7)	SUA predicted progression of CKD only in unadjusted analysis	No
Weiner (2008)	13,338 (57.4)	USA; healthy	Prospective cohort (8.5)	Each 1 mg/dL increase in SUA increased CKD risk by 7–11%	Yes
Hsu (2009)	177,570 (40.7)	USA; healthy	Prospective cohort (median 25.7)	Higher quartile of SUA conferred 2.14-fold increased risk of ESRD	Yes
Madero (2009)	840 (52)	USA; CKD 3,4	Retrospective cohort (median 10)	SUA correlated with death but not ESRD	No
See (2009)	28,745 (40.8)	Taiwan; healthy	Prospective cohort (7)	SUA > 7.7 mg/dL in men and >6.6 mg/dL in women only weakly associated with prevalent renal impairment	Yes
Bellomo (2010)	900 (43.1)	Italy; healthy	Prospective cohort (5)	Each 1 mg/dL increase in SUA correlated with 28% increased risk of reduced eGFR in 5 years	Yes
Ben Dov (2011)	2,449 (48)	Israel; healthy	Prospective cohort (26)	SUA >6.5 mg/dL in men and >5.3 mg/dL in women associated with 2.1-fold increased risk of CKD	Yes
Yamada (2011)	14,399 (49.1)	Japan; healthy	Prospective cohort (5)	Each 1 mg/dL increase in SUA increased risk of newly diagnosed CKD (42% in men, 32% in women)	Yes
Dawson (2013)	6,984 (50.3)	UK; healthy	Prospective cohort (median 29 in men and 34 in women)	Highest quartile of SUA associated with GFR decline	Yes

Table 1. Continued

Author (year)	Participants (mean age, years)	Country; at risk	Design (follow-up, years)	Finding on SUA and kidney function	Statistical significance
Iseki (2013)	16,630	Japan; healthy	Prospective cohort (10)	Increased SUA within normal range predicted eGFR decline over 10 years	Yes
Chang (2015)	701 (62.3)	Japan; eGFR 30-60; T2DM, CGN, HT	Retrospective cohort (median 4.5)	Baseline SUA nor time-averaged SUA over 2 years did not confer an independent effect on ESRD	No
Kuriyama (2015)	8,223 (39)	Japan; healthy	Prospective cohort (4)	SUA was not chosen as an independent estimate to predict the incident CKD in this multivariate analysis adjusted for eGFR and male	No
Yan (2015)	3,212 (61.0)	China; T2DM	Cross-section	SUA was an independent predictor of diabetic kidney disease	Yes
Uchida (2015)	803 (63)	Japan; eGFR 15-60; T2DM, CGN, HT	Retrospective cohort (median 4.0), propensity score analysis	Propensity score analysis showed the effect of SUA <6.5 mg/dL in the follow-up on the incidence of ESRD	Yes
Rodenbach (2015)	627 (12.3)	USA; CKD children	Prospective cohort (5)	Hyperuricemia was an independent risk factor for faster progression of CKD in children and adolescents	Yes

CKD, chronic kidney disease; SUA, serum uric acid; ESRD, end stage renal disease; HR, hazard ratio; eGFR, estimated glomerular filtration rate; T2DM, type 2 diabetes mellitus; CGN, chronic glomerulonephritis; HT, hypertension.

gression only when the analysis was not adjusted for baseline kidney function parameters. After adjusting for baseline GFR and proteinuria, hyperuricemia was no longer a risk factor of CKD progression [26]. Likewise, post hoc analysis of the Modification of Diet in Renal Disease study enrolling 838 patients with stage 3–4 CKD showed that hyperuricemia was associated with an increased risk of all-cause mortality and cardiovascular disease mortality but not with kidney failure [27]. In addition, certain Japanese cohorts did not show the independent significance of the effect of SUA on the incidence of CKD over the 4-year observation period [25] (Table 1).

Recently we analyzed the cohort data by a propensity score method to clarify the independent impact of SUA on the subsequent risk of ESRD [28]. A retrospective CKD cohort was used (n = 803). After propensity score matching, the higher SUA showed elevated hazard ratios (HRs) by Kaplan-Meier analysis (≥6.0 mg/dL, HR 4.53, 95% CI 1.79–11.43; ≥6.5 mg/dL, HR 3.39, 95% CI 1.55–

Table 2. Randomized controlled trials using urate-lowering drugs on CKD (cited from ref [25])

Author (published year)	Country; at risk (*n*) follow-up, y or m	Drug, dosage per day	Finding on kidney function
Siu (2006)	China; SCr 1.35–4.50 mg/dL (54); 1 year	Allopurinol, 100–300 mg	slowed progression of CKD
Kanbay (2007)	Turkey; eGFR >60 ml/min (69); 3 months	Allopurinol, 300 mg	increased eGFR from 79 to 92 mL/min
Goicoechea (2010)	Spain; CKD 3 (113); 2 years	Allopurinol, 100 mg	slowed decline in eGFR
Momeni (2010)	Iran; T2DM (SCr <3.0 mg/dL) (40); 4 months	Allopurinol, 100 mg	reduced proteinuria
Kanbay (2011)	Turkey; CKD 2 (97); 4 months	Allopurinol, 300 mg	increased eGFR from 86 to 90 mL/min
Pai (2013)	India; CKD 3,4 (183); 2 years	Allopurinol, 100 mg	reduced blood pressure and progression of CKD
Goicoechea (2015)	Spain; CKD 3 (113); 7 years	Allopurinol, 100 mg	inhibited the incidence of renal outcome
Sircar (2015)	India; CKD 3, 4 (93); 6 months	Febuxostat, 40 mg	slowed the decline in eGFR

y, years; m, months; SCr, serum creatinine; CKD, chronic kidney disease; eGFR, estimated glomerular filtration rate.

7.42; ≥7.0 mg/dL, HR 2.19, 95% CI 1.28–3.75). To our surprise, the number needed to treat was estimated to be as small as 8 to 9 over 5 years. From our study, SUA should be targeted at less than 6.0 mg/dL [28].

Effects of Urate Lowering Therapy on CKD in Randomized Controlled Trials

Since SUA may be an important risk factor for the progression of renal dysfunction, hypertension, and lifestyle-related diseases such as metabolic syndrome or T2DM, lowering SUA may represent a new therapeutic venue. The clinical trials of SUA-lowering therapy published until now are listed in Table 2.

Allopurinol

Several studies have investigated the treatment effect of the XO inhibitor allopurinol on renal outcomes [21, 29–32]. Recent meta-analyses, however, have produced inconsistent results. In a meta-analysis of 8 randomized controlled trials (RCTs), allopurinol had no effect on estimated GFR compared with controls in 5 trials ($n = 346$) but abrogated increases in serum creatinine in 3 trials ($n = 130$) [33]. Allopurinol had no effect on proteinuria and data for effects of allopurinol on progression to ESRD were scant. In another meta-analysis of 19 RCTs enrolling 992 patients with stage 3–5 CKD, allopurinol significantly reduced SUA levels and blood pressure, and with more favorable eGFR compared with controls [34]. There was appreciable heterogeneity among the trials regarding study design, duration of follow-up and baseline kidney function in both meta-analyses. Moreover, there is the possibility that the favorable results by allopurinol may be related to effects other than lowering SUA levels. XO produces reactive oxygen species (ROS) and inhibition of this ROS formation by allopurinol may have some renoprotective effects [20, 34].

Febuxostat

Febuxostat is a novel XO inhibitor and used with safety in the patients with kidney dysfunction. In a recent report of RCT of 93 patients with CKD stage 3 and 4 (45 patients in febuxostat and 48 in placebo), febuxostat slowed the decline in eGFR compared to placebo [35]. The mean eGFR in the febuxostat group showed a nonsignificant increase from a baseline of 31.5 ± 13.6 to 34.7 ± 18.1 mL/min/1.73 m^2 at 6 months. With placebo, mean eGFR decreased from 32.6 ± 11.6 to 28.2 ± 11.5 mL/min/1.73 m^2 ($p = 0.003$). Seventeen of 45 (38%) participants in the febuxostat group had >10% decline in eGFR over baseline compared with 26 of 48 (54%) from the placebo group ($p < 0.004$) [35]. However, the sample size of this study is small and duration of follow-up is very short. Therefore, an ongoing study of a larger sample size and longer duration is expected to elucidate the role of UA-lowering drug in the clinical setting [36].

Conclusions

The hypothesis that SUA is a possible mediator of the progression of kidney diseases has a history of more than a century. Over the past decade, basic research and clinical studies suggested that the elevation of SUA may directly deteriorate the structure and function of the healthy kidney and that hyperuricemia may be a target of treatments of CKD. Although recent intervention studies using UA-lowering drugs showed promising results of delaying CKD progression, the results are far from conclusive. Larger and well-designed RCTs of UA-lowering therapy will be warranted to assess the precise renoprotective effects of the therapy.

Acknowledgments

We thank all of the doctors at the Division of Nephrology, Teikyo University School of Medicine, Tokyo, Japan, for their cooperation. This work was supported in part by a Grant-in-Aid for Progressive Renal Diseases Research on Rare and Intractable Disease, from the Ministry of Health, Labour and Welfare of Japan (to SU) and Gout Research Foundation (to SU) and JSPS KAKENHI grants 16K00871 (to SU). The funders had no role in making the decision to publish and prepare this manuscript.

Disclosure Statement

The authors have declared that no competing interests exist.

References

1 Yang W, Xie D, Anderson AH, Joffe MM, Greene T, Teal V, Hsu CY, Fink JC, He J, Lash JP, Ojo A, Rahman M, Nessel L, Kusek JW, Feldman HI: Association of kidney disease outcomes with risk factors for CKD: findings from the Chronic Renal Insufficiency Cohort (CRIC) study. Am J Kidney Dis 2014;63:236–243.

2 Johnson RJ, Nakagawa T, Jalal D, Sanchez-Lozada LG, Kang DH, Ritz E: Uric acid and chronic kidney disease: which is chasing which? Nephrol Dial Transplant 2013;28:2221–2228.

3 Yano H, Tamura Y, Kobayashi K, Tanemoto M, Uchida S: Uric acid transporter ABCG2 is increased in the intestine of the 5/6 nephrectomy rat model of chronic kidney disease. Clin Exp Nephrol 2014;18:50–55.

4 Nagura M, Tamura Y, Kumagai T, Hosoyamada M, Uchida S: Uric acid metabolism of kidney and intestine in a rat model of chronic kidney disease. Nucleosides Nucleotides Nucleic Acids 2016; 35:550–558.

5 Chino Y, Samukawa Y, Sakai S, Nakai Y, Yamaguchi J, Nakanishi T, Tamai I: SGLT2 inhibitor lowers serum uric acid through alteration of uric acid transport activity in renal tubule by increased glycosuria. Biopharm Drug Dispos 2014;35:391–404.

6 Toyoki D, Shibata S, Kuribayashi-Okuma E, Xu N, Ishizawa K, Hosoyamada M, Uchida S: Insulin stimulates uric acid reabsorption via regulating urate transporter 1 and 1 ATP-binding cassette sub-family G member 2. Am J Physiol Renal Physiol 2017;313:F826–F834.

7 See LC, Kuo CF, Chuang FH, Li HY, Chen YM, Chen HW, Yu KH: Serum uric acid is independently associated with metabolic syndrome in subjects with and without a low estimated glomerular filtration rate. J Rheumatol 2009;36:1691–1698.

8 Kanbay M, Jensen T, Solak Y, Le M, Roncal-Jimenez C, Rivard C, Lanaspa MA, Nakagawa T, Johnson RJ: Uric acid in metabolic syndrome: from an innocent bystander to a central player. Eur J Intern Med 2016;29:3–8.

9 Sanchez-Lozada LG, Lanaspa MA, Cristobal-Garcia M, Garcia-Arroyo F, Soto V, Cruz-Robles D, Nakagawa T, Yu MA, Kang DH, Johnson RJ: Uric acid-induced endothelial dysfunction is associated with mitochondrial alterations and decreased intracellular ATP concentrations. Nephron Exp Nephrol 2012; 121:e71–e78.

10 Chen C-Y, Lv JM, Yao QZ: Hyperuricemia-related diseases and xanthine oxidoreductase (XOR) inhibitors: an overview. Med Sci Monit 2016;22:2501–2512.

11 Kang DH, Nakagawa T, Feng L, Watanabe S, Han L, Mazzali M, Truong L, Harris R, Johnson RJ: A role for uric acid in the progression of renal disease. J Am Soc Nephrol 2002;13:2888–2897.

12 Mazzali M, Hughes J, Kim YG, Jefferson JA, Kang DH, Gordon KL, Lan HY, Kivlighn S, Johnson RJ: Elevated uric acid increases blood pressure in the rat by a novel crystal-independent mechanism. Hypertension 2001; 38:1101–1106.

13 Nakagawa T, Mazzali M, Kang DH, Kanellis J, Watanabe S, Sanchez-Lozada LG, Rodriguez-Iturbe B, Herrera-Acosta J, Johnson RJ: Hyperuricemia causes glomerular hypertrophy in the rat. Am J Nephrol 2003;23:2–7.

14 Jalal DI, Maahs DM, Hovind P, Nakagawa T: Uric acid as a mediator of diabetic nephropathy. Semin Nephrol 2011;31:459–465.
15 Sanchez-Lozada LG, Tapia E, Santamaria J, Avila-Casado C, Soto V, Nepomuceno T, Rodriguez-Iturbe B, Johnson RJ, Herrera-Acosta J: Mild hyperuricemia induces vasoconstriction and maintains glomerular hypertension in normal and remnant kidney rats. Kidney Int 2005;67:237–247.
16 Ryu ES, Kim MJ, Shin HS, Jang YH, Choi HS, Jo I, Johnson RJ, Kang DH: Uric acid-induced phenotypic transition of renal tubular cells as a novel mechanism of chronic kidney disease. Am J Physiol Renal Physiol 2013; 304:F471–480.
17 Kosugi T, Nakayama T, Heinig M, Zhang L, Yuzawa Y, Sanchez-Lozada LG, Roncal C, Johnson RJ, Nakagawa T: Effect of lowering uric acid on renal disease in the type 2 diabetic db/db mice. Am J Physiol Renal Physiol 2009;297:F481–F488.
18 Diamond JR, Bonventre JV, Karnovsky MJ: A role for oxygen free radicals in aminonucleoside nephrosis. Kidney Int 1986;29:478–483.
19 Kawamorita Y, Shiraishi T, Tamura Y, Kumagai T, Shibata S, Fujigaki Y, Hosoyamada M, Nakagawa T, Uchida S: Renoprotective effect of topiroxostat via antioxidant activity in puromycin aminonucleoside nephrosis rats. Physiol Rep 2017;5. pii: e13358.
20 Kang DH, Chen W: Uric acid and chronic kidney disease: new understanding of an old problem. Semin Nephrol 2011;31:447–452.
21 Mende C: Management of chronic kidney disease: the relationship between serum uric acid and development of nephropathy. Adv Ther 2015;32:1177–1191.
22 Li L, Yang C, Zhao Y, Zeng X, Liu F, Fu P: Is hyperuricemia an independent risk factor for new-onset chronic kidney disease?: a systematic review and meta-analysis based on observational cohort studies. BMC Nephrol 2014; 15:122.
23 Yan D, Tu Y, Jiang F, Wang J, Zhang R, Sun X, Wang T, Wang S, Bao Y, Hu C, Jia W: Uric Acid is independently associated with diabetic kidney disease: a cross-sectional study in a Chinese population. PLoS One 2015;10:e0129797.
24 Testa A, Mallamaci F, Spoto B, Pisano A, Sanguedolce MC, Tripepi G, Leonardis D, Zoccali C: Association of a polymorphism in a gene encoding a urate transporter with CKD progression. Clin J Am Soc Nephrol 2014;9:1059–1065.
25 Kumagai T, Ota T, Tamura Y, Chang WX, Shibata S, Uchida S: Time to target uric acid to retard CKD progression. Clin Exp Nephrol 2017;21:182–192.
26 Sturm G, Kollerits B, Neyer U, Ritz E, Kronenberg F: Uric acid as a risk factor for progression of non-diabetic chronic kidney disease? The Mild to Moderate Kidney Disease (MMKD) Study. Exp Gerontol 2008;43:347–352.
27 Madero M, Sarnak MJ, Wang X, Greene T, Beck GJ, Kusek JW, Collins AJ, Levey AS, Menon V: Uric acid and long-term outcomes in CKD. Am J Kidney Dis 2009;53:796–803.
28 Uchida S, Chang WX, Ota T, Tamura Y, Shiraishi T, Kumagai T, Shibata S, Fujigaki Y, Hosoyamada M, Kaneko K, Shen ZY, Fujimori S: Targeting uric acid and the inhibition of progression to end-stage renal disease-a propensity score analysis. PLoS One 2015; 10:e0145506.
29 Siu YP, Leung KT, Tong MK, Kwan TH: Use of allopurinol in slowing the progression of renal disease through its ability to lower serum uric acid level. Am J Kidney Dis 2006;47: 51–59.
30 Kanbay M, Ozkara A, Selcoki Y, Isik B, Turgut F, Bavbek N, Uz E, Akcay A, Yigitoglu R, Covic A: Effect of treatment of hyperuricemia with allopurinol on blood pressure, creatinine clearance, and proteinuria in patients with normal renal functions. Int Urol Nephrol 2007;39:1227–1233.
31 Goicoechea M, de Vinuesa SG, Verdalles U, Ruiz-Caro C, Ampuero J, Rincon A, Arroyo D, Luno J: Effect of allopurinol in chronic kidney disease progression and cardiovascular risk. Clin J Am Soc Nephrol 2010;5:1388–1393.
32 Goicoechea M, Garcia de Vinuesa S, Verdalles U, Verde E, Macias N, Santos A, Perez de Jose A, Cedeno S, Linares T, Luno J: Allopurinol and progression of CKD and cardiovascular events: long-term follow-up of a randomized clinical trial. Am J Kidney Dis 2015; 65:543–549.

33 Bose B, Badve SV, Hiremath SS, Boudville N, Brown FG, Cass A, de Zoysa JR, Fassett RG, Faull R, Harris DC, Hawley CM, Kanellis J, Palmer SC, Perkovic V, Pascoe EM, Rangan GK, Walker RJ, Walters G, Johnson DW: Effects of uric acid-lowering therapy on renal outcomes: a systematic review and meta-analysis. Nephrol Dial Transplant 2014;29: 406–413.
34 Kanji T, Gandhi M, Clase CM, Yang R: Urate lowering therapy to improve renal outcomes in patients with chronic kidney disease: systematic review and meta-analysis. BMC Nephrol 2015;16:58.
35 Sircar D, Chatterjee S, Waikhom R, Golay V, Raychaudhury A, Pandey R: Efficacy of febuxostat for slowing the GFR decline in patients with CKD and asymptomatic hyperuricemia: a 6-month, double-blind, randomized, placebo-controlled trial. Am J Kidney Dis 2015;66:945–950.
36 Hosoya T, Kimura K, Itoh S, Inaba M, Uchida S, Tomino Y, Makino H, Matsuo S, Yamamoto T, Ohno I, Shibagaki Y, Iimuro S, Imai N, Kuwabara M, Hayakawa H: The effect of febuxostat to prevent a further reduction in renal function of patients with hyperuricemia who have never had gout and are complicated by chronic kidney disease stage 3:study protocol for a multicenter randomized controlled study. Trials 2014;15:26.

Shunya Uchida, MD, PhD
Department of Internal Medicine, Teikyo University School of Medicine
2–11–1 Kaga, Itabashi-ku
Tokyo 173–8605 (Japan)
E-Mail s_uchida@netjoy.ne.jp

Treviño-Becerra A, Iseki K (eds): Uric Acid in Chronic Kidney Disease.
Contrib Nephrol. Basel, Karger, 2018, vol 192, pp 69–76 (DOI: 10.1159/000484280)

Uric Acid: The Lower the Better?

Gianni Bellomo · Antonio Selvi

Department of Nephrology, USL 1 Regione Umbria, Perugia, Italy

Abstract

Background: Uric acid (UA) is still considered a risk factor, or even a causative agent, for chronic kidney disease (CKD); however, a few, important, clinical questions remain unanswered; in particular: when and whether urate-lowering therapy should be commenced in subjects with asymptomatic hyperuricemia and/or monosodium urate crystals deposition? What is the most appropriate UA target to be achieved and how long does it need to be maintained? How does treatment need be adjusted in patients with chronic kidney disease? ***Summary:*** The observational and intervention studies available do not fully answer such questions, and a treatment to target trial is required. We provide here some preliminary opinion on how such a trial might be designed. A final unresolved issue relates to the possible (if any) dangers of overtreatment of hyperuricemia, leading to "hypouricemia," which may occur more frequently with newer, more potent, drugs. A U- or J-shaped association has been found between UA levels and mortality in epidemiologic studies; patients with congenital hypouricemia are more prone to exercise-induced renal failure; a theoretical concern, linked to more complete Xanthine Oxidase inhibition, may involve xanthine nephropathy, although up to now, it has been observed almost exclusively in patients with tumor lysis syndrome. ***Key Messages:*** Although there is no definite answer to the title question at the moment, available information tends to indicate a treatment target with serum UA levels between 5.0 and 6.0 mg/dL as reasonable.

Introduction

A role for uric acid (UA) in the pathogenesis and progression of renal disease had been proposed almost a century ago, however, it was too hastily dismissed in the early eighties. A body of evidence, mostly accumulated during the last decade [1–3], has led to a reappraisal of the influence of UA on hypertension, cardiovascular, and renal disease in particular. At present, however, it is not known when and whether to commence urate-lowering therapy in subjects with asymptomatic hyperuricemia and/or monosodium urate crystals deposition, what is the most appropriate UA target to be achieved, and how long does it need to be maintained and how does treatment need be modulated in patients with chronic kidney disease(CKD). Answers to such questions have been tentatively provided for patients with gout: in fact, the EULAR most recent guidelines [4] suggest that in patients on urate-lowering treatment, serum UA level should be monitored and maintained to <6.0 mg/dL (360 mmol/L). A lower serum UA target (<5.0 mg/dL; 300 mmol/L) to facilitate faster dissolution of crystals is recommended for patients with severe gout (tophi, chronic arthropathy, frequent attacks) until total crystal dissolution and resolution of gout, based on the fact that a number of studies have shown that treating to an UA target lower than 6.0 mg/dL (monosodium urate crystal deposition in tissues occurs at a concentration greater than 6.8 mg/dL) results in the reduction of incident gout flares, as well as shrinkage and dissolution of tophi [5]. Such information is not available for asymptomatic patients and the role of UA in the so-called non-gout diseases, CKD in particular, is uncertain and cannot be definitely established by observational studies. In this case, what we really need is a treatment to target trial, comparing prospectively the renal benefits (if any) achieved at different UA targets.

A Treatment to Target Trial of Hyperuricemia

Table 1 proposes a crude outline of how such a study could be designed, only to be intended as a stimulus for further discussion. In fact, a number of issues arise in dealing with such a trial: the definition of asymptomatic uricemia itself is far from being unequivocally established [6, 7], as it could be statistical-laboratory (serum UA >2 standard deviations above the mean for healthy population), based on physiology (the in vivo urate saturation concentration at which crystals begin to form), or the risk of developing disease, which is largely unknown. A further point to be clarified relates to the size of the sample, as it is likely for women to be underrepresented; in addition, should different targets be considered for women? A degree of cross-over between groups is to be expected; thus, the choice of using the "intention to treat as a primary analysis"; subgroup analysis should include Xanthin Oxidase (XO) inhibitors compared to other hypouricemic drugs, to rule out an effect of XO inhibition per se, and debatably, men and women. Finally, we propose to study an essentially healthy (aside from hyperuricemia) population, as we believe it to be the only effective way to exclude confounding by other risk factors for CKD.

Table 1. Proposed outline of a treatment to target trial of asymptomatic hyperuricemia

Study population: subjects with asymptomatic hyperuricemia (>7.0 mg/dL)
Age: 18–65 years
Normal baseline renal function
Normotensive, non-diabetics, no gout, not treated with hypouricemic drugs and/or diuretics, normoalbuminuria
Randomized to one of three arms: No specific urate-lowering intervention Urate-lowering treatment to target serum UA <6.0 mg/dL Urate-lowering treatment to target serum UA <4.0 mg/dL
Target may be achieved with any of the following: XOi, uricosuric agents, uricases, diet, other
Duration of the study: 5 years, with yearly visits for renal function and UA determinations
Primary outcome measure: eGFR change(CKD-EPI) vs. baseline
Secondary outcome measures: eGFR slope, incident hypertension, incident diabetes, new onset albuminuria, incident CKD, incident CV events, side effects
Analysis: intention to treat (primary), per protocol (secondary), adjusted for baseline e-GFR. Missing data handled by the Last Observation Carried Forward (LOCF) approach
Subgroup analysis: XOi/non-XOi hypouricemic agents Men/women?

What do we expect from such a trial? Ideally, if serum UA targets were achieved, if estimated glomerular filtration rate were better preserved in the treatment groups and more so in the lower serum UA arm, if estimated glomerular filtration rate change were comparable in subjects treated with XO inhibitors and other hypouricemic agents, we might be able to conclude that UA is indeed a renal risk factor and that lowering its levels provides renal benefits proportional to the degree of its lowering, not attributable to XO inhibition per se.

Up to now, we have been dealing with the realm of fantasy and wishful thinking.

In reality (facts), there are only a few randomized controlled trials of hypouricemic treatment [8–16], briefly outlined in Table 2. These trials are quite heterogeneous regarding population studied (mostly patients with CKD), intervention (mostly allopurinol or febuxostat), duration of the study, use of placebo, outcome measures (eGFR change, proteinuria, blood pressure, incident CKD, "hard" renal events). Despite such heterogeneity, all the available investigations tend to agree toward a beneficial effect of lowering serum UA, as in-

Table 2. Summary of available trials of hyperuricemia treatment

Author (ref)	Country, year	Population, *n*	Intervention	Duration of study	Outcome	sUA (mg/dL start → end of study
Siu [8]	Taiwan, 2006	CKD 3–4, *n* = 54	Allopurinol 100–300 mg vs. usual therapy	1 year	reduced BP, slowing serum creatinine increase	Intervention: 9.75 → 5.88 Control: 9.92 → 10.08
Momeni [9]	Iran, 2010	type 2 DM with nephropathy (proteinuria + serum creatinine <3.0 mg/dL, *n* = 40)	Allopurinol 100 mg vs. placebo	4 months	reduction of proteinuria in intervention group	Intervention: 5.96 → 5.31 Placebo: 6.50–6.44
Goicoechea [10]	Spain, 2010	CKD 3, *n*=113	Allopurinol 100 mg vs. placebo	2 years	slowing of eGFR decline	Intervention: 7.8 → 6.0 Placebo: 7.3 → 7.5
Goicoechea [11]	Spain, 2015	CKD 3, *n* = 113	Allopurinol 100 mg vs. placebo	7 years	slowing of eGFR decline, reduced incidence of renal events	Intervention: 7.8 → 6.6 Placebo: 7.3→ 7.1
Kanbay [12]	Turkey, 2011	Asymptomatic hyperuricemia, *n* = 97	Allopurinol 300 mg vs. no treatment	4 months	reduced BP, increased eGFR in allopurinol group	Intervention: 8.3 → 5.8 Control: 7.9 → 7.2
Santhosh Pai [13]	India, 2013	CKD, stage 3–4, *n* = 183	allopurinol 100 mg vs. no treatment	2 years	reduction of blood pressure and CKD progression in treated group	Intervention: 9.1 → 5.3 Control: 9.2 → 9.9
Sircar [14]	India, 2015	CKD 3–4, *n* = 93	febuxostat 40 mg vs. placebo	6 months	slowing of eGFR decline in febuxostat group	Intervention: 9.0 → 5.2 Placebo: 8.2 → 7.8
Weng [15]	Taiwan, 2016	CKD, *n* = 2,460	febuxostat "ab initio" (*n* = 40), conversion to febuxostat from other (oULT *n* = 206), vs. oULT continued, *n* = 2,214	1 year	slowing of eGFR decline in febuxostat and conversion groups compare to oULT	Febuxostat: 9.5–6.7 Conversion: 8.5 → 6.3 oULT: 7.2→7.0
Krishnamurthy [16]	USA, 2017	Hyperuricemia, *n* = 100, males	Allopurinol, 200 mg, average, vs no treatment	3.4 years	Lower adjusted creatinine in allopurinol group	Allopurinol: 9.2 → 6.4 Control: 8.7 → 8.9

dicated by a recent meta-analysis and a systematic review [17, 18]. It must be observed, though, that in some studies, blood pressure was also reduced; thus, it is not clear whether the renal effect was due to serum UA lowering, reduced blood pressure, or both. Despite the heterogeneity of the intervention studies, a beneficial renal effect was achieved at an average serum UA level consistently above 5.0, and often 6.0 mg/dL; so, from a renal standpoint, there is no compelling evidence to overtreat hyperuricemia, and given the results of the intervention studies, a target serum UA between 5.0 and 6.0 mg/dL, appears to be sufficient.

Two ongoing studies are likely to provide important results in the near future; one study performed in type 1 diabetics (allopurinol vs placebo), namely, the Preventing Early Renal Loss in Diabetes study [19], involved centers located in the United States, Canada, Denmark, was of 3 years duration, and the primary outcome measure of this study was the change in i (iohexol-determined) GFR. The other [20] study called the FREED (Febuxostat for Cerebral and Cardiorenovascular Events Prevention Study) of 3 years duration, investigated an elderly Japanese population (febuxostat vs allopurinol), with any one of the following primary outcomes: a composite of cerebral, cardiovascular, and renal events, and all deaths including death due to cerebral, cardiovascular, and renal disease, new or recurring cerebrovascular disease, new or recurring non-fatal coronary artery disease, cardiac failure requiring hospitalization, arteriosclerotic disease requiring treatment, renal impairment, new atrial fibrillation, and all deaths other than cerebral or cardiovascular or renal disease.

Overtreatment of Hyperuricemia: When is Low Too Low?

In recent years, the advent of new potent hypouricemic drugs has led to the possibility of intensifying treatment, and it is not uncommon to see patients with serum UA levels below 3.0 or even 2.0 mg/dL. Actually it is not known whether hypouricemia is harmful or at which concentration should serum UA be considered to be too low. Hypouricemia, usually defined as serum UA <2.0 mg/dL, is asymptomatic. Pregnant women may show serum UA <3.0 or even <2.0 mg/dL, with no apparent harm to the mother or fetus. Congenital hypouricemia with hyperuricosuria may result from a number of defects in urate transporters. Such patients are more often asymptomatic; however, they may be more prone to develop renal failure following strenuous exercise, as well as urate lithiasis [21]. Most epidemiological studies show a J-shaped relation between UA levels and CV morbidity and mortality: in a study from Taiwan

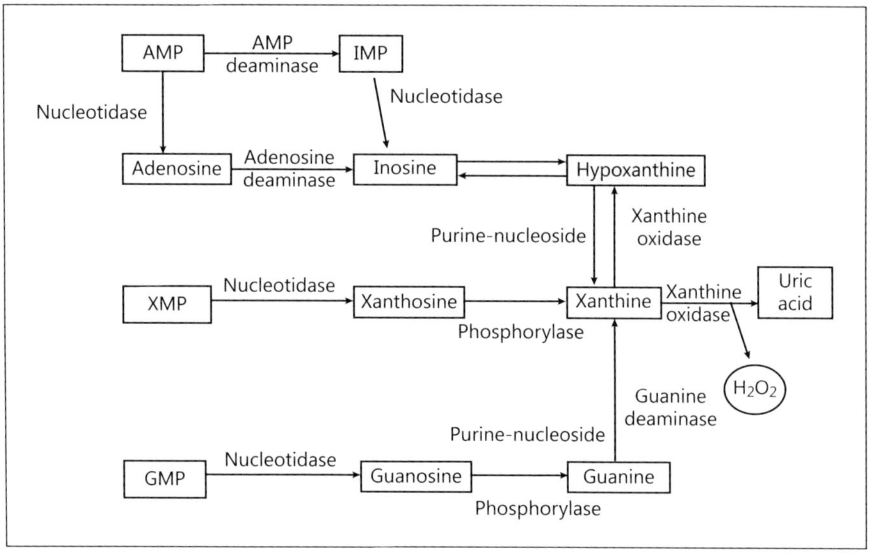

Fig. 1. Purine catabolism in man.

[22], CV hazard was demonstrated to rise steeply with increasing serum UA (particularly in heart failure), but a moderate increase was apparent also for very low serum UA. Another study [23] performed in hemodialysis patients showed all-cause mortality to increase in the lowest and highest serum UA quintiles. A study performed in patients with stage 5 CKD [24] confirmed a J-shaped association between serum UA levels and all-cause mortality, which was shown to increase both in the higher and lower serum UA quintiles. It must be borne in mind, however, that the hypouricemia observed in epidemiological studies most likely results from malnutrition [25] rather than being a consequence of pharmacological (over) treatment. Conversely, in treated patients, serum UA is also a marker of the extent of XO inhibition; with increasing blockage of XO, precursor compounds (Fig. 1) such as hypoxanthine (highly soluble, poses no problems) and xanthine (insoluble at physiologic pH) tend to accumulate. A theoretical concern about the risk of developing xanthine nephropathy may exist: a few cases, limited to patients with the tumor lysis syndrome, have been reported with the use of allopurinol [26], but we do not know whether the use of more potent, non-competitive XO inhibitors may increase such a risk. In addition, in rats, xanthine crystals induced by topiroxostat, a novel, potent XO inhibitor, have been shown to cause transitional cell tumors [27].

Finally, in patients with gout, the EULAR guidelines [4] suggest that serum UA lower than 3.0 mg/dL is not recommended in the long term.

Conclusions

A definitive answer to the title question (UA and the Kidney, the Lower the Better?) is not available and requires a treatment to target trial of hyperuricemia; however, to our knowledge, no such trial has been completed yet. The few, heterogeneous, randomized controlled trials available have consistently shown beneficial effects on renal function with treatment of hyperuricemia; such effects are achieved at average serum UA levels >5.0 mg/dL and often >6.0 mg/dL, so, a target serum UA between 5.0 and 6.0 mg/dL appears reasonable. Although hypouricemia in itself does not seem to pose a threat to the patients' health, there are potential concerns of overtreatment and it is recommended to avoid long-term serum UA levels <3.0 mg/dL.

References

1 Jalal DI, Chonchol M, Chen W, Targher G: Uric acid as a target in CKD. Am J Kidney Dis 2012;61:134–146.
2 Johnson RJ, Nakagawa T, Jalal D, Sanchez-Losada LG, Kang DH, Ritz E: Uric acid and chronic kidney disease: which is chasing which? Nephrol Dial Transplant 2013;28:2221–2228.
3 Bellomo G: Uric acid and chronic kidney disease: a time to act? World J Nephrol 2013;2:17–25.
4 Richette P, Doherty M, Pascual E, et al: 2016 updated EULAR evidence-based recommendations for the treatment of gout. Ann Rheum Dis 2017;76:29–42.
5 Ruoff G, Edwards NL: Overview of serum uric acid treatment targets in gout: why less than 6 mg/dL? Postgrad Med 2016;128:706–715.
6 Bardin T, Richette P: Definition of hyperuricemia and gouty conditions. Curr Opin Rheumatol 2014;26:186–191.
7 Stamp K, Dalbeth N: Urate-lowering therapy for asymptomatic hyperuricemia: a need for caution. Sem Arhritis Rheumatism 2017;46:457–464.
8 Siu YP, Leung KT, Tong MKA, Kwan TH: Use of Allopurinol in Slowing the Progression of Renal Disease Through Its Ability to Lower Serum Uric Acid Level. Am J Kidney Dis 2006;47:51–59.
9 Momeni A, Shahrzad S, Seirafian S, Taheri S, Kheiri S: Effect of allopurinol in decreasing proteinuria in type 2 diabetic patients. IJKD 2010;4:128–132.
10 Goicoechea M, Garcia-Vinuesa MS, Verdalles U, et al: Effect of allopurinol in chronic kidney disease (CKD) progression and cardiovascular risk. Clin J Am Soc Nephrol 2010;5:1388–1393.
11 Goicoechea M, Garcia de Vinuesa S, Verdalles U, et al: Allopurinol and progression of CKD and cardiovascular events: long-term follow-up of a randomized clinical trial. Am J Kidney Dis 2015;65:543–549.
12 Kanbay M, Huddam B, Azak A, et al: A randomized study of allopurinol on endothelial function and estimated glomerular filtration rate in asymptomatic hyperuricemic subjects with normal renal function. Clin J Am Soc Nephrol 2011;6:1887–1994.
13 Pai BH, Swarnalatha G, Ram R, Dakshinamurty KV: Allopurinol for prevention of progression of kidney disease with hyperuricemia. Indian J Nephrol 2013;23:280–286.
14 Sircar D, Chatterjee S, Waikhom R, Golay V, Raychaudhury A, Chatterjee S, Pandey R: Efficacy of febuxostat for slowing the GFR decline in patients with CKD and asymptomatic hyperuricemia: a 6-month, double-blind, randomized, placebo-controlled trial. Am J Kidney Dis 2015;66:945–950.

15 Weng SC, Tarng DC, Chen YC, Wu MJ: Febuxostat is superior to traditional urate-lowering agents in reducing the progression of kidney function in chronic kidney disease patients. Cogent Med 2016;3:1213–1215.
16 Krishnamurty A, Lazaro D, Stefanov DG, Blumenthal D, Gerber D, Patel S: The effect of allopurinol on renal function. J Clin Rheumatol 2017;23:1–5.
17 Xia X, Luo Q, Li B, Lin Z, Yu X, Huang F: Serum uric acid and mortality in chronic kidney disease: a systematic review and meta-analysis. Metabolism 2017;65:1326–1341.
18 Kumagai T, Ota T, Tamura Y, Chang WX, Shibata S, Uchida S: Time to target uric acid to retard CKD progression. Clin Exp Nephrol 2017;21:182–192.
19 The PERL (Preventing Early Renal Loss in Diabetes) Study. www.perl-study.org.
20 Kojima S, Matsui K, Ogawa H, et al: Rationale, design, and baseline characteristics of a study to evaluate the effect of febuxostat in preventing cerebral, cardiovascular, and renal events in patients with hyperuricemia. J Cardiol 2017;69:169–175.
21 Sebesta I: Genetic disorders resulting inhyper- or hypouricemia. Adv Chronic Kidney Dis 2012;19:398–403.
22 Kuo CF, See LC, Yu KH, Chou iJ, Chiou MJ, Luo SF: Significance of serum uric acid levels on the risk of all-cause and cardiovascular mortality. Rheumatology (Oxford) 2013;52: 127–134.
23 Hsu SP, Pai MF, Peng YS, Chiang CK, Ho TI, Hung KY: Serum uric acid levels show a "J-shaped"_association with all-cause mortality in haemodialysis patients. Nephrol Dial Transplant Nephrol Dial Transplant 2004;19: 457–462.
24 Suliman ME, Johnson RJ, García-López E, Qureshi AR, et al: J-shaped mortality relationship for uric acid in CKD. Am J Kidney Dis 2006;48:761–771.
25 Park C, Obi Y, Streja E, Rhee CM, Catabay CJ, Vaziri ND, Kovesdy CP, Kalantar-Zadeh K: Serum uric acid, protein intake and mortality in hemodialysis patients. Nephrol Dial Transplant 2017;32:1750–1757.
26 LaRosa C, McMullen L, Bakdash S, Ellis D, Krishnamurti L, Wu HY, Moritz ML: Acute renal failure from xanthine nephropathy during management of acute leukemia. Pediatr Nephrol 2007;22:132–135.
27 Shimo T, Moto M, Ashizawa N, Matsumoto K, Iwanaga T, Saito K: Xanthine crystals induced by topiroxostat, a xanthine oxidoreductase inhibitor, in rats, cause transitional cell tumors. Arch Toxicol 2014;88:1035–1042.

Gianni Bellomo, MD
Department of Nephrology, USL 1 Regione Umbria, Perugia, MVT Hospital
Via del Buda
IT–06059 Todi (Italy)
E-Mail Gianni.bellomo@uslumbria1.it

Treviño-Becerra A, Iseki K (eds): Uric Acid in Chronic Kidney Disease.
Contrib Nephrol. Basel, Karger, 2018, vol 192, pp 77–81 (DOI: 10.1159/000484281)

Gout: A Disease of Kings

Sydney C.W. Tang

Division of Nephrology, Department of Medicine, The University of Hong Kong, Hong Kong, China

Abstract

As a disease of kings, and the king of diseases, gout is one of the oldest joint diseases known to humans. First described as far back as 2640 B.C., gout is still the most common form of inflammatory arthritis haunting humans in the 21st century. The disease is caused by the chronic elevation of serum uric acid levels above the saturation point for monosodium urate crystal formation. Its incidence is progressively rising even today, but there are also regional and ethnic variations. Finally, the role of genetics is only beginning to be unraveled.

Historical Perspective

Gout has been hailed "A disease of kings, the king of diseases." It was first identified by the Egyptians in approximately 2640 B.C. Hippocrates of Kos (c. 460–c. 370 B.C.) was a Greek physician often referred to as the Father of Western Medicine, described gout in the fifth century B.C. as the "unwalkable disease," a condition of older men and a product of high living. The term gout originated from the Lain word "gutta" meaning a drop, as the ancient belief has it that the devil causes the disease by instilling a poisonous humor into the joint of the victim drop by drop.

Sir Alfred Baring Garrod (1819–1907) was an English physician who obtained his medical doctorate at the University College Hospital of London in 1843. Five years later, in 1848, he had discovered an abnormally high uric acid level in the blood of patients with gout, and correctly identified uric acid as the cause of gout and not the effect of gout. He was the first to propose using lithium as a remedy for the disorder. As he also recommended lithium as a treatment for mental illness, he hypothesized that gout could be a cause of mood disorders such as mania and depression. He is also credited for coining the term "rheumatoid arthritis."

In 1969, McCarty and Hollander [1] proved the association between acute arthritis in gout and deposition of uric acid crystals in the joints. In 1988, Sir James Black (also from the University College Hospital), Gertrude Elion and George Hitchings shared in Nobel Prize in Physiology or Medicine for their discoveries of important principles for drug treatment of this condition.

Uric Acid Evolution and Primitive Cultures

Early hominoids live in tropical rain forests where fruits (fructose) are the main source of food. The earth went from the Oligocene through the Miocene and into the Pliocene as it cooled into a series of ice ages, leading to food shortage.

The Miocene warming began 21 million years ago and continued until 14 million years ago, when global temperatures took a sharp drop – the Middle Miocene Climate Transition (MMCT). Early hominoids (Apes) ancestors on very low sodium diet (0.5 g/day compared with an average of 8–10 g/day today).

Urate production culminates in the final steps of purine metabolism. Most mammals synthesize uricase to further convert the less-soluble urate into the more water-soluble allantoin. During the MMCT, it was found that a loss of function mutation in the uricase gene led to elevated blood pressure and salt sensitivity. The survival advantage helped maintain blood pressure during environmental stress.

Mammals that possess uricase had serum uric acid levels of 0.5–2 mg/dL, whereas apes lacking uricase had serum uric acid levels in the range of 2.5–3.5 mg/dL (Fig. 1) [2]. The progressive loss of uricase activity allowed our ancestors to readily accumulate fat via the metabolism of fructose from fruits. This adaptation provided our ancestors with an advantage when the energy-rich rainforests of Europe and Asia were displaced by temperate forests by the end of the Oligocene.

Epidemiology

There is a wide variation in the prevalence of gout in various populations. The prevalence of gout is >1% in most developed countries, especially in North America and Europe. Epidemiological evidence from the United States, the

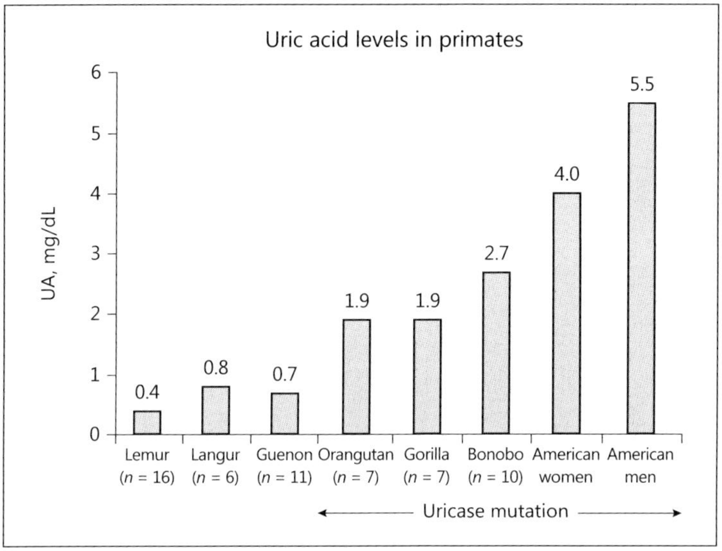

Fig. 1. Differences in serum uric acid levels in different primates.

United Kingdom, New Zealand, and China suggests that gout is becoming more prevalent. In the United States, the prevalence of gout in a managed-care administrative claims database increased from 2.9/1,000 in 1990 to 5.2/1,000 in 1999. The National Health and Nutrition Examination Survey 2007–2008 determined that 3.9% of the adult population (age ≥20 years) in the United States had self-reported gout over the period 2007–2008 [3]. In the United Kingdom, the prevalence of gout from surveys undertaken in general practice diagnostic indices increased from 2.6/1,000 in 1975, 3.4/1,000 in 1987, to 9.5/1,000 in 1993 [4].

In Asia, the ethnic groups in Malaysia and China such as Malays and Tamils have higher uric acid levels compared to other populations in the continent. In comparison with Caucasians, Japanese have much lower uric acid levels. The prevalence of gouty arthritis in Thailand is low [5]. Worldwide, the highest reported frequency of gout is from the modern Pacific Islander populations. Both Maori and European males in New Zealand have a very high prevalence of gout [6]. Compared to European females, Polynesian women have much higher serum uric acid levels.

In India, females have a later onset, longer duration, and higher uric acid levels as against the males. Polyarticular gout was more frequent in the elderly and females, with a greater association with tophi, renal involvement, and ischemic heart disease. Hypertension, diabetes, and obesity were more frequent in oligoarticular gout [7].

Taiwan is another country with the highest prevalence of gout. Taiwanese aborigines have a very high prevalence of gout, which is shared with their genetically related Polynesian cousins, the Maori and indigenous Oceania – Pacific Islander populations [8]. A recent study using the National Health Insurance Research Database found an incidence of 2.74/1,000 person-years in 2010 and that the incidence decreased throughout the period from 2005 to 2010 [9].

Genetics

Clinical and epidemiological evidence as well as recent advances in genetic studies suggest that a genetic component contributes to the development of gout. The varying prevalence of gout as highlighted above suggests ethnic and genetic differences. This is also supported by the existence of familial aggregation of gout [10]. In addition, a migration study reported a ninefold increase in the risk of gout in Tokelauan migrants living in urban New Zealand compared with non-migrants, highlighting the gene-environment interaction in the occurrence of gout [11].

Genome-wide association studies (GWASs) in the 2000s have identified single nucleotide polymorphisms in genes encoding transporters involved in renal and gut clearance of uric acid [12]. For instance, the high frequencies of renal urate transporter SLC2A9 haplotypes (GLUT9) associated with susceptibility to gout have been reported in modern Maori and Pacific Islanders in New Zealand [13]. This genetic abnormality marked reduces uric acid excretion. Unlike SLC2A9, ABCG2 is found to have a strong effect only in people of western Polynesian ancestry [14].

To date, the most comprehensive GWAS, published in 2013, combined data from more than 140,000 individuals of European ancestry and identified and replicated 28 loci associated with serum urate [15]. Of note, all these currently known associations account only for 7% of the variance in serum uric acid levels, implying a large as yet unidentified gap between known specific genetic associations and the demonstrated heritability of hyperuricemia.

Conclusions

This review on the historical, epidemiologic, and genetic aspects of gout suggests that while this disease has been with humans for as long as we have existed, a lot of unknowns still exist. The marked regional variation in gout prevalence, as well as the paucity of reliable data on the incidence of gout in many parts of the world is but one area of deficiency. Ethnic background and genetic makeup clearly affect gout prevalence and support a considerable contribution of genetic factors to gout. The search for candidate genes that influence serum uric acid levels has provided only rudimentary evidence of specific genetic polymorphisms that are associated with the risk of gout, but a large proportion of the demonstrated heritability of gout remains unexplained. Given that gout is a common complex disorder, variation in the mix of gene-environment interaction poses great challenges to the study of gout epidemiology and genetics.

References

1 McCarty DJ, Hollander JL: Identification of urate crystals in gouty synovial fluid. Ann Intern Med 1961;54:452–460.
2 Johnson RJ, Titte S, Cade JR, Rideout BA, Oliver WJ: Uric acid, evolution and primitive cultures. Semin Nephrol 2005;25:3–8.
3 Zhu Y, Pandya BJ, Choi HK: Prevalence of gout and hyperuricemia in the US general population: the National Health and Nutrition Examination Survey 2007–2008. Arthritis Rheum 2011;63:3136–3141.
4 Harris CM, Lloyd DC, Lewis J: The prevalence and prophylaxis of gout in England. J Clin Epidemiol 1995;48:1153–1158.
5 Lohsoonthorn V, Dhanamun B, Williams MA: Prevalence of Hyperuricemia and its relationship with metabolic syndrome in Thai adults receiving annual health exams. Arch Med Res 2006;37:883–889.
6 Gibson T, Waterworth R, Hatfield P, Robinson G, Bremner K: Hyperuricaemia, gout and kidney function in New Zealand Maori men. Br J Rheumatol 1984;23:276–282.
7 Porkodi R, Parthipan M, Rukmangatharajan S, et al: Clinical spectrum of gout in South India. J Indian Rheumatol Assoc 2002;10:61–63.
8 Chang SJ, Ko YC, Wang TN, et al: High prevalence of gout and related risk factors in Taiwan's Aborigines. J Rheumatol 1997;24:1364–1369
9 Kuo CF, et al: Epidemiology and management of gout in Taiwan: a nationwide population study. Arthritis Res Ther 2015;17:13.
10 Kuo CF, et al: Familial aggregation of gout and relative genetic and environmental contributions: a nationwide population study in Taiwan. Ann Rheum Dis 2015;74:369–374.
11 Prior IA, Welby TJ, Ostbye T, Salmond CE, Stokes YM: Migration and gout: the Tokelau Island migrant study. Br Med J (Clin Res Ed) 1987;295:457–461.
12 Obermayr RP, et al: Elevated uric acid increases the risk for kidney disease. J Am Soc Nephrol 2008;19:2407–2413.
13 Hollis-Moffatt JE, Xu X, Dalbeth N, et al: Role of urate transporter SLC2A9 gene in susceptibility to gout in New Zealand Māori, Pacific Island and Caucasian case-control sample sets. Arthritis Rheum 2009;60:3485–3492.
14 Phipps-Green AJ, Hollis-Moffatt JE, Dalbeth N, Merriman M, et al: A strong role for the ABCG2 gene in susceptibility to gout in New Zealand Pacific Island and Caucasian, but not Māori, case and control sample sets. Hum Mol Genet 2010;19:4813–4819.
15 Köttgen A, et al: Genome-wide association analyses identify 18 new loci associated with serum urate concentrations. Nat Genet 2013;45:145–154.

Sydney Tang
Department of Medicine, The University of Hong Kong
Rm 415, Professorial Block, Queen Mary Hospital
102 Pokfulam Road
Hong Kong (China)
E-Mail scwtang@hku.hk

Treviño-Becerra A, Iseki K (eds): Uric Acid in Chronic Kidney Disease.
Contrib Nephrol. Basel, Karger, 2018, vol 192, pp 82–87 (DOI: 10.1159/000484282)

Systemic Implications of Hyperuricemia

Juan A. Tamayo y Orozco

Senior professor – Head of the Renal Health Area in the Academic Secretariat from the National Institute of Public Health, S.S.A. Member of the National Academy of Medicine, Mexico City, Mexico

Abstract

Systemic implications of hyperuricemia need to be reconsidered in the context of the energy and protein wasting being an early indicator of organ deterioration in patients affected by the cardiometabolic syndrome and other frequent pathology states like preeclampsia, hyperparathyroidism, and chronic renal failure. This chapter points out physiological alterations that are to be made related to hyperuricemia, new diagnostic strategies, and early therapeutic interventions in the context of the old enemy: asymptomatic hyperuricemia. This chapter also concludes with a proposal to undertake research in this emerging, primary care, cost-efficient scenario.

Introduction

Abnormalities in the metabolism of uric acid (UA), namely, over ingestion of precursors, metabolic over production, and lower rates of clearance from our body lead to the accumulation of this molecule in system fluids and tissues [1]. This triggers several reactions, highly dependent on hydrogen-ion concentration, from simple crystallization in joints and tissues, to chronic and severe inflammation, and derangements of the endothelium, leading to thrombosis, fibrosis, and tissue/organ deterioration and faster progression of disease. Such is the case of chronic kidney disease evolution – it invariably ends in renal failure [1–10].

Therefore, it is important to consider UA (the final product of purine and pyrimidine utilization, guanine, and adenine) abnormalities in the metabolic context as a whole, considering its role in altering nitrogen balance in the body not only in the clinical and epidemiological context of its cardio-metabolic repercussions, in organ-specific damage such as kidney, and cardiovascular disease but also in physiological states like pregnancy.

Nitrogen is a fuel for protein synthesis, including nucleotides and nucleic acids. Its utilization is highly dependent on energy production and consumption. This implies the proportion in which fat and carbohydrates are simultaneously used in the intermediary metabolism: they represent the most important energy sources for a healthy life [1, 11, 12].

Therefore, in the day-to-day clinical practice, the early detection of the triggering and development of the "Protein and Energy Wasting syndrome" (PEW) is becoming very relevant [13]. PEW is being more carefully included as an influential factor associated with the development of many of the noncommunicable chronic degenerative diseases. These in turn are increasing the global burden of cardio-metabolic outcomes, which are challenging most of our health systems worldwide. Such is the case of myocardial, cerebral infractions, and chronic renal diseases [13–16].

The purpose of this collaboration is to call for the importance of the primary-care attention of UA abnormalities; permanent or recurrent, hyper or hypouricemic states, as a simple measurable marker of derangements in nitrogen and energy utilization of our circadian, intermediate metabolism [17–20].

Consequently, the presence of UA abnormalities must lead to a careful evaluation of well-described mechanisms leading to PEW. Of these, even mild metabolic or respiratory acidosis plays a key role in very common clinical scenarios like cardio-metabolic syndrome, diabetes mellitus, pregnancy, hyperparathyroidism, urinary stone disease, overweight, and obesity (to mention only a few, analyzed elsewhere in this book). Designing clinical interventions focused to prevent and avoid the development of PEW must be associated with better, cost-efficient, and optimal quality outcomes. UA abnormalities must be considered an early and sensitive marker of such clinical conditions [9, 18–20].

Clinical Approach

From the clinical point of view, measuring UA concentration in serum is feasible even in the more rudimentary primary care system. This fact, favors the possibility of alerting the primary health team to consider minimal but repeated deviations of UA concentrations in a patient as a warning signal of early endothelial damage.

It is proposed that finding ≥5 mg/dL of UA in plasma of women and ≥6 mg/dL in men (both within the normal reference values for most laboratories) should alert the clinician (most likely a general practitioner) to initiate an assessment of systemic inflammation. The initial steps must include correlating the UA concentration with urea/creatinine ratio, serum albumin, CO_2, and some systemic inflammation markers like: globular sedimentation rate, C-reactive protein, or homocysteine in all patients with cardio-metabolic syndromes, associated or not, with overweight and/or obesity [1, 10, 18].

Abnormal and persistent UA elevations, or finding a ≤3 mg/dL UA blood concentration in both genders [18] combined with ≥20 urea/creatinine, ≤3 g/L serum albumin, total venous CO_2 ≤20 mEq/L, a very active globular sedimentation rate, high C-reactive protein or homocysteine, are criteria to establish the clinical suspicion of PEW [10]. Thus, more careful evaluation and optimal intervention, including both of nutrition and either a specific or generic medication are required.

This is a novel challenge and there are no clinical guidelines or any consensus that has been published at this early stage of UA abnormality identification. The fact is, that with new evidence emerging from epidemiological studies from Japan [9] and the growing evidence of metabolic pathways involved in the evolution of the PEW syndrome, this initiative is appealing because it may be very effective and feasible in the primary care setting [21–25].

The nutritional strategies to be implemented in the early stages of PEW are more readily feasible than those required with more advanced metabolic alterations. They must be less restrictive and simple to adopt in the day-to-day life of a patient with cardio-metabolic risk [22, 25]. The availability of keto-analogues of essential amino acids may be very useful to reintegrate nitrogen to protein, perform nucleotide synthesis, and to improve the proteasome-ubiquitin complex [22]. The use of SGLPT2 and ABCG2 blockers is also a very important and novel option to clear UA from our body and to get the additional benefits of losing weight and gaining better control of arterial blood pressure. In diabetic patients, a better control of carbohydrate and fat metabolism is achieved [26, 27] in addition to folic acid supplementation [28].

When the intervention measures just described are started early in the evolution of diabetic syndrome, they may delay the appearance of early markers of kidney endothelial, podocyte, tubular (KIM 1), or interstitial damage (NGCL, IGF β receptor isoforms 1, 2, and 3). Therefore, it is important to allow the clinician to initiate nephron-protection and systemic organ preservation at a stage where clinical outcomes may be more successful than what is currently being done: interventions are started when there is a 40% reduction in nephron number, estimated glomerular filtration rate is just 60%, and there is prevalence of microalbuminuria. This may be too late to achieve stabilization and it is less likely to obtain the reversal of the already deteriorated kidney functional reserve.

A similar scenario would be coronary and carotid/intracerebral endothelial health, allowing the primary-care system to refer these cases to a program specialized in the management of these frequent but not standardized conditions. Contemporary clinical guidelines do not include UA abnormalities as a marker for early diagnosis and hence, more opportune interventions, which may result in better clinical outcomes [8, 24].

This challenging proposal is supported by all the contributions of this publication and requires serious analysis and urgency to arrive at a consensus.

Conclusions

As more evidence is accumulated, it is becoming evident that UA is an early marker of nitrogen and energy wasting from our body. Values considered normal previously may not be so currently. It is proposed that a slight but persistent elevation of UA associated with abnormal urea/creatinine ratio, low serum concentration of carbon dioxide (CO_2) and one or more systemic inflammation markers, must lead to a serious diagnostic evaluation in a person with one or more of the conditions included in the diagnosis of cardio-metabolic syndrome (especially dyslipidemia, any type of diabetes mellitus, and arterial hypertension with overweight/obesity).

Establishing an initial phase of PEW must allow effective, low-cost, and optimal-outcome interventions. The role of inhibitors of the SGLPT2 receptor in the proximal renal tubule as well as a rational use of keto-and hydroxy analogues of essential amino acids, with folic acid may be additional resources to be considered and studied in special case conditions.

Research is needed in this emerging, primary care, cost-efficient proposal.

References

1 Maiuolo J, Oppedisano F, Gratteri S, Muscoli C, Mollace V: Regulation of uric acid metabolism and excretion. Int J Cardiol 2016;213: 8–14.

2 Zha Y, Qian Q: Protein nutrition and malnutrition in CKD and ESRD. Nutrients 2017; 9:pii:E208.

3 Suzuki M, Masakane I, Nakajima M, Ito S, Seino Y, Yabuki K: Protein nenrgy wasting (pew) is subclinically progressive in choronic dialysis patients. Kidney Res Clin Pract 2012; 31:A77.

4 Agnelli S: Regulation of amino acid catabolism in rats fed diets with different protein content. Universitat de Barcelona, Barcelona, Spain, 2016.

5 Gu L, Huang L, Wu H, Lou Q, Bian R: Serum uric acid to creatinine ratio: a predictor of incident chronic kidney disease in type 2 diabetes mellitus patients with preserved kidney function. Diab Vasc Dis Res 2017;14:221–225.
6 Lecker SH, Solomon V, Mitch WE, Goldberg AL: Muscle protein breakdown and the critical role of the ubiquitin-proteasome pathway in normal and disease states. J Nutr 1999; 129(1S suppl):227S–237S.
7 Beddhu S, Chen X, Wei G, Raj D, Raphael KL, Boucher R, Chonchol MB, Murtaugh MA, Greene T: Associations of protein-energy wasting syndrome criteria with body composition and mortality in the general and moderate chronic kidney disease populations in the United States. Kidney Int Rep 2017;2: 390–399.
8 Eleftheriadis T, Golphinopoulos S, Pissas G, Stefanidis I: Asymptomatic hyperuricemia and chronic kidney disease: narrative review of a treatment controversial. J Adv Res 2017; 8:555–560.
9 Nagahama K, Inoue T, Kohagura K, Kinjo K, Ohya Y: Associations between serum uric acid levels and the incidence of hypertension and metabolic syndrome: a 4-year follow-up study of a large screened cohort in Okinawa, Japan. Hypertens Res 2015;38: 213–218.
10 Rymarz A, Bartoszewicz Z, Szamotulska K, Niemczyk S: The associations between body cell mass and nutritional and inflammatory markers in patients with chronic kidney disease and in subjects without kidney disease. J Ren Nutr 2016;26:87–92.
11 Sakuma K (ed): The plasticity of skeletal muscle. From molecular mechanism to clinical applications. Singapore, Springer, 2017.
12 Beddhu S, Wei G, Chen X, Boucher R, Kiani R, Raj D, Murtaugh MA: Associations of dietary protein and energy intakes with protein-energy wasting syndrome in hemodialysis patients KI reports (May). 2017. https://doi.org/10.1016/j.ekir.2017.04.002.
13 Leitner LM, Wilson RJ, Yan Z, Gödecke A: Reactive oxygen species/nitric oxide mediated inter-organ communication in skeletal muscle wasting diseases. Antioxid Redox Signal 2017;26:700–717.
14 Wang YW, Lin TY, Peng CH, Huang JL, Hung SC: Factors associated with decreased lean tissue index in patients with chronic kidney disease. Nutrients 2017;9:pii:E434.
15 Kiuchi A, Ohashi Y, Tai R, Aoki T, Mizuiri S, Ogura T, Aikawa A, Sakai K: Association between low dietary protein intake and geriatric nutrition risk index in patients with chronic kidney disease: A retrospective single-center cohort study. Nutrients 2016; 8:pii:E662.
16 Noce A, Vidiri MF, Marrone G, Moriconi E, Bocedi A, Capria A, Rovella V, Ricci G, De Lorenzo A, Di Daniele N: Is low-protein diet a possible risk factor of malnutrition in chronic kidney disease patients? Cell Death Discov 2016;2:16026.
17 Vargas-Santos AB, Neogi T: Management of gout and hyperuricemia in CKD. Am J Kidney Dis 2017;70:422–439.
18 Bae E, Cho HJ, Shin N, Kim SM, Yang SH, Kim DK, Lee H: Lower serum uric acid level predicts mortality in dialysis patients. Medicine (Baltimore) 2016;95:e3701.
19 Tsai CW, Lin SY, Kuo CC, Huang CC: Serum uric acid and progression of kidney disease: a longitudinal analysis and mini-review. PLoS One 2017;12:e0170393.
20 Snelson M, Clarke RE, Coughlan MT: Stirring the pot: can dietary modification alleviate the burden of CKD? Nutrients 2017; 9:pii:E265.
21 Moorthi RN, Avin KG: Clinical relevance of sarcopenia in chronic kidney disease. Curr Opin Nephrol Hypertens 2017;26:219–228.
22 Dickinson JM, Reidy PT, Gundermann DM, Borack MS, Walker DK, D'Lugos AC, Volpi E, Rasmussen BB: The impact of postexercise essential amino acid ingestion on the ubiquitin proteasome and autophagosomal-lysosomal systems in skeletal muscle of older men. J Appl Physiol 2017;122: 620–630.
23 Marcelli D, Brand K, Ponce P, Milkowski A, Marelli C, Ok E, et al: Longitudinal changes in body composition in patients after initiation of hemodialysis therapy: results from an international cohort. J Ren Nutr 2016;26:72–80.
24 Ramirez MEG, Bargman JM: Treatment of asymptomatic hyperuricemia in chronic kidney disease: a new target in an old enemy – a review. J Adv Res 2017;8:551–554.

25 Iseki K, Yamagata K: A practical approach of salt and protein restriction for CKD patients in Japan. BMC Nephrol 2016;17:87.
26 Davies MJ, Trujillo A, Vijapurkar U, Damaraju CV, Meininger G: Effect of canagliflozin on serum uric acid in patients with type 2 diabetes mellitus. Diabetes Obes Metab 2015;17:426–429.
27 Miyata H, Takada T, Toyoda Y, Matsuo H, Ichida K, Suzuki H: Identification of febuxostat as a new strong ABCG2 inhibitor: potential applications and risks in clinical situations. Front Pharmacol 2016;7:518.
28 Scheepers LE: Folic acid: the solution for treating asymptomatic hyperuricemia? Am J Clin Nutr 2017;105:775–776.

Prof. Juan A. Tamayo y Orozco
Accessalud, Insurgentes Sur Av. 299
Ph. Col.condesa, del. Cuauhtemoc
06100 Ciudad de México (Mexico)
E-Mail dr.tamayo@accessalud.com

Treviño-Becerra A, Iseki K (eds): Uric Acid in Chronic Kidney Disease.
Contrib Nephrol. Basel, Karger, 2018, vol 192, pp 88–102 (DOI: 10.1159/000484283)

Uric Acid as a Cause of the Metabolic Syndrome

Christopher King[a] • Miguel A. Lanaspa[a] • Thomas Jensen[a] • Dean R. Tolan[b] • L. Gabriela Sánchez-Lozada[c] • Richard J. Johnson[a]

[a]Division of Renal Diseases and Hypertension, University of Colorado Denver, Aurora, CO, and [b]Department of Biology, Boston University, Boston, MA, USA; [c]Laboratory of Renal Physiopathology, INC Ignacio Chávez, Mexico City, Mexico

Abstract

Hyperuricemia is common in subjects with obesity, metabolic syndrome, and type 2 diabetes. For many years, hyperuricemia was attributed to the effects of insulin resistance to reduce urinary excretion of uric acid, and it was believed that uric acid may not have any causal role in the metabolic syndrome. However, in recent years, hyperuricemia has been found to independently predict the development of diabetes. Experimental studies have also shown that hyperuricemia may mediate insulin resistance, fatty liver, and dyslipidemia in both fructose-dependent and fructose-independent models of metabolic syndrome. The mechanism for uric acid-induced insulin resistance appears to be mediated by the development of mitochondrial oxidative stress and impairment of insulin-dependent stimulation of nitric oxide in endothelial cells. Pilot studies in humans have reported a potential benefit of lowering serum uric acid on insulin resistance. Large clinical trials are recommended. If uric acid is shown to be a mediator of incident type 2 diabetes in humans, then lowering serum uric acid would represent a simple and inexpensive way to help prevent the development of diabetes and to slow the epidemic.

The recognition by Lancereaux in 1880 that there were two types of diabetes mellitus, with one associated with obesity and the other with wasting and weight loss [1] was also accompanied by parallel observations that the "obese"

Dr. Christopher King's (Deceased) work was part of an affiliation with the Renal Division of the University of Colorado.

presentation of diabetes was also commonly accompanied by gout [2, 3]. Indeed, by the early 1920s, it was recognized that a condition of prediabetes was common in which subjects would have mildly elevated blood glucose levels, systemic hypertension, obesity, and hyperuricemia [4]. By the 1960s and 1970s, the association of uric acid with prediabetes and type 2 diabetes was well documented [5–10], and as the metabolic syndrome (syndrome X) became recognized as an entity [11], so was hyperuricemia recognized as an accompanying sign [12].

However, most studies suggested that the hyperuricemia was a consequence of reduced renal excretion of uric acid due to the effects of hyperinsulinemia [13] or due to reduced kidney function that accompanied the diabetic state, and there was little thought that hyperuricemia had a role in the pathogenesis of obesity or the prediabetic state. Indeed, hyperuricemia is not considered a key component of the metabolic syndrome, nor is it usually measured as a biomarker for diabetic risk.

In this chapter, we review the burgeoning evidence that hyperuricemia itself may have a contributory or causal role in the pathogenesis of insulin resistance and diabetes.

Metabolic Syndrome: A Form of Fat Storage

The metabolic syndrome is recognized as a constellation of signs that include an "abdominal" pattern of obesity with increased body waist circumference, dyslipidemia associated with high serum triglycerides and low HDL cholesterol, elevated blood pressure, and impaired glucose tolerance (manifested as a type of insulin resistance). Other commonly associated characteristics include nonalcoholic fatty liver disease, microalbuminuria, and hyperuricemia. While the constellation of signs is well recognized, the clinical importance of recognizing the syndrome has been challenged because some studies suggest that the syndrome does not carry any greater cardiovascular risk than its individual components [14–17]. Indeed, Reaven, who helped champion the recognition of the syndrome, later felt that it provided minimal additional prognostic information for cardiovascular disease than the use of the classical Framingham risk score and that it did not predict diabetes any better than simply using the fasting plasma glucose [18].

However, whether or not it carries any better prognostic role than individual components of the syndrome does not necessarily detract from its potential importance as a syndrome with a common pathogenic basis. Indeed, by evaluating other animals that have found means for storing fat in preparation for periods of food shortage, such as long-distance migrating birds [19] and hibernating mammals [20, 21], it has been understood that all of the signs of metabolic syndrome represent the normal physiological response for storing fuel and that it should be renamed "fat storage syndrome" [22]. Indeed, the syndrome could be viewed as a protective mechanism in which the animal stores fat (in the form of adipose, fatty liver, and elevated serum triglycerides), which leads to low-grade inflammation in blood and tissues (muscle, fat, liver) leading to insulin resistance. Mild insulin resistance augments fuel metabolism to promote primarily the use of free fatty acids with glucose being reserved for use by the brain and maintain redox reactions. In addition, there are increases in blood pressure to help maintain perfusion of its organs.

The etiology of the fat storage syndrome has been an area of major interest, with focus being on the causes of obesity and insulin resistance. At the basis has been the recognition that leptin resistance is a feature resulting in an impaired satiety response [23] and that there is commonly impairment in hepatic and skeletal muscle fatty acid oxidation [24]. Endothelial dysfunction may play a role [25] and more recently, there has also been some evidence that vasopressin may have some partial role [26, 27].

Role of Fructose in Metabolic Syndrome

One of the strongest risk factors for the development of metabolic syndrome is the intake of sugary beverages [28, 29]. Refined sugar (or sucrose) consists of a disaccharide of glucose and fructose and is similar in composition to high fructose corn syrup, which consists of a mixture of glucose and fructose monosaccharides. The administration of fructose to mice and rats can rapidly re-create the metabolic syndrome, especially if the sugars are administered in the drinking water.

Studies suggest that both the fructose and glucose component can induce obesity, fatty liver, and insulin resistance when administered in the drinking water. However, the fructose component is especially effective to induce weight gain, as it can induce leptin resistance and stimulate increased food intake, and also block fatty acid oxidation in the liver. While much of the weight gain is from the hyperphagia that results even when food intake is controlled such that both fructose- and sugar-fed animals ingest the same number of calories as the control group eating glucose (or starch), there are significant differences [30–32]. Indeed, significant detrimental effects on blood pressure, fatty liver, serum triglycerides, and insulin resistance will tend to develop in the fructose-fed animals compared to the control group, even though there is no difference in final weights [14–17]. Similar studies in humans also show that fructose preferentially causes visceral fat accumulation, dyslipidemia, decreased insulin sensitivity, impaired postprandial fat oxidation, and reduced resting energy expenditure compared to glucose [33–35].

The administration of glucose in the drinking water can also induce features of metabolic syndrome associated with hyperphagia and weight gain. However, studies suggest that a significant component of the weight gain, fatty liver, and hyperinsulinemia is due to the conversion of glucose to fructose in the body due to the activation of the polyol (aldose reductase-sorbitol dehydrogenase) pathway. Indeed, if fructose metabolism is blocked (by utilizing fructokinase knockout mice), then glucose-fed animals still get fat but show fewer features of metabolic syndrome [36].

Fructose and Uric Acid: Activation of AMP Deaminase

One of the striking findings is that fructose is the only commonly ingested carbohydrate that generates uric acid during its metabolism [37, 38]. This is due to the presence of fructokinase C, an enzyme present in the intestine, liver, and kidney, as well as in other sites such as the islets, adipose tissue, hippocampus, and hypothalamus [39–41]. Fructokinase C causes such rapid phosphorylation of fructose to fructose 1-phosphate that intracellular ATP, GTP, and phosphate levels fall, leading to AMP accumulation [37, 38, 42]. The fall in intracellular GTP and phosphate activates the enzyme AMP deaminase [43] as does the accumulation of fructose 1-phosphate [44]. IMP levels increase [42], which along with GMP are metabolized to generate uric acid. In turn, uric acid inhibits AMP-activated protein kinase, thus promoting more AMP to be metabolized by AMP deaminase [44, 45], while also further stimulating both the generation of fructose via effects on aldose reductase [46] and by the stimulation of fructose metabolism by increasing fructokinase expression and activity [47]. In addition, the accumulation of IMP, GDP, and GMP inhibits the enzyme aldolase B, further potentiating fructokinase activity and stimulation of the turnover of ATP (Fig. 1) [42]. As uric acid continues to accumulate, xanthine oxidase becomes inhibited [48, 49] but likely at the expense of continued upstream activation of the AMP deaminase pathway.

Following ingestion of fructose, uric acid rapidly accumulates within the cell, increasing tenfold or more [50]. Serum uric acid then rises, peaking 15–30 min after ingestion [51, 52]. In humans, postprandial increases in serum uric

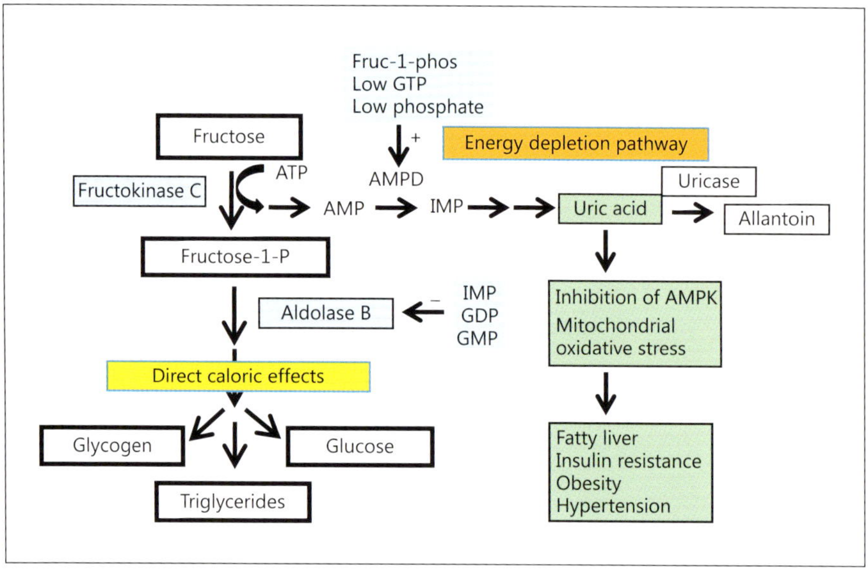

Fig. 1. Possible mechanism for fructose-mediated fatty liver and insulin resistance. Fructose is metabolized by fructokinase C that generates fructose-1-phosphate, which is then further metabolized via classical caloric pathways to generate ATP and glucose, glycogen, and triglycerides. However, the initial phosphorylation of fructose is associated with rapid intracellular phosphate, GTP, and ATP depletion that leads to AMP accumulation and activation of AMP deaminase. In addition, the accumulation of IMP, GDP, and GMP inhibit the enzyme aldolase B, further potentiating fructokinase activity and stimulation of the turnover of ATP (Fig. 1). The generation of uric acid is associated with both mitochondrial oxidative stress and inhibition of AMP-activated protein kinase (AMPK), which are responsible for causing many of the effects of fructose leading to induce metabolic syndrome.

acid can be observed following fructose-rich meals [53]. Chronic high intake of fructose is also associated with a tendency for higher fasting serum uric acid levels [54].

Role of Uric Acid in Fructose-Dependent and -Independent Models of Metabolic Syndrome

The observation that uric acid could have proinflammatory [55, 56] and pro-oxidative [57, 58] effects, and that it could induce endothelial dysfunction [59], raised the possibility that it might have a role in insulin resistance-metabolic syndrome. Indeed, we found that lowering serum uric acid with either a xanthine oxidase inhibitor (allopurinol or febuxostat), or with the uricosuric, benzbromarone, could reduce features of the metabolic syndrome in the fructose-fed rat [30, 60]. Benefits could be observed not only on blood pressure but also on serum triglycerides, insulin resistance, and fatty liver [30, 31, 47, 60]. Baldwin et al. [61] also studied the pound mouse, a mouse with a leptin receptor defect that develops hyperuricemia and severe metabolic syndrome. In these mice, the use of allopurinol blocked inflammation (macrophage infiltration) in the fat tissue prevented the decrease in adipose and circulating adiponectin, and improved blood pressure and insulin resistance [61]. Some reduction in hepatic fat was also observed [62].

Human Studies on the Role of Uric Acid in Metabolic Syndrome and Diabetes

Epidemiological studies have reported a strong association of obesity and metabolic syndrome in subjects with gout and/or hyperuricemia [63, 64]. More importantly, an elevated serum uric acid has been found to independently predict the development of obesity, metabolic syndrome, nonalcoholic fatty liver disease, and diabetes in multiple studies [65–83]. Hyperuricemia is also a potent independent predictor of hypertension [84, 85].

There are limited studies evaluating the effect of lowering uric acid on insulin resistance. Several studies in humans have reported that allopurinol [86–88], or benzbromarone [89], can improve insulin resistance in subjects with metabolic syndrome. In addition, another study showed that allopurinol reduced markers of liver inflammation and with improvement in lipids in patients with nonalcoholic fatty liver disease compared to placebo [90]. However, another study was unable to show an improvement in insulin resistance in subjects administered high-dose fructose [91]. All of these were small pilot studies, and it is evident that large clinical trials need to be performed. In addition, while there are small pilot studies showing some improvement in blood pressure in subjects with metabolic syndrome [92, 93], further studies are needed before any definitive conclusions can be drawn.

Potential Mechanisms by Which Fructose and Uric Acid May Induce Insulin Resistance, Fatty Liver, and High Blood Pressure

Studies by Sanchez-Lozada et al. [94, 95] have shown that the hypertensive response to hyperuricemia is mediated by oxidative stress and endothelial dysfunction, and Mazzali et al. [96, 97] also showed a clear role for activation of the renin angiotensin system. Similarly, oxidative stress is also the underlying mechanism by which uric acid induces inflammation in adipocytes [61, 98] and hepatocytes [62, 99]. The observation that uric acid can induce oxidative stress in cells may appear surprising, as uric acid is known as an antioxidant that can inactivate superoxide anion, hydroxyl radical, and peroxynitrite [100, 101]. However, uric acid can also be a prooxidant and can generate oxidants (triuretcarbonyl radical and aminocarbonyl radical) on reaction with peroxynitrite [102, 103], and urate hydroperoxides on reaction with myeloperoxidase and hydrogen peroxide [104, 105].

However, most of the oxidative stress that appears is due to the stimulation of NOX4-expressing NADPH oxidase [62, 98, 99, 106]. In liver-derived cells, Nox4 translocates to the mitochondrial outer membrane following uric acid exposure, resulting in NADPH oxidase-dependent mitochondrial oxidative stress [62, 99] as well as rotenone-sensitive oxidative stress due to the activity of mitochondrial complex 1 of the respiratory chain [99]. A precedent for NOX4-associated NADPH oxidase in mitochondria has been reported by others where it has been thought to be important in the pathogenesis of diabetes [107, 108].

The mitochondrial oxidative stress induced by uric acid has been shown in the hepatocyte to contribute to both lipogenesis and impaired fatty acid oxidation [44, 62]. The former occurs due to the inhibition of aconitase, with the accumulation of citrate that enters into the cystosol and stimulates ATP citrate lyase and lipogenesis [62]. The oxidative stress also inactivates enoyl CoA hydratase, resulting in a blockade of fatty acid oxidation [44]. A uric acid inhibition of AMP-activated protein kinase also occurs, which then stimulates gluconeogenesis and further impairs fatty acid oxidation [44, 45]. Mitochondrial oxidative stress in endothelial cells also results in an impairment of insulin-dependent nitric oxide release, impairing glucose delivery to the periphery [109]. All of these effects help mediate the metabolic phenotype.

We have also postulated ("the Chris King hypothesis") that the oxidants generated in the mitochondrial could result in the release of hydrogen peroxide (generated by mitochondrial superoxide dismutase) that leaves the mitochondria via aquaporin 8 [110, 111] and, in the cytosol, oxidizes phosphorylated Akt2 on Cys124, causing reduced translocation of GLUT4 and insulin resistance [112].

Supporting these observations is the consistent finding that both fructose and uric acid can induce mitochondrial oxidative stress, that the fructose-dependent mitochondrial oxidative stress can be reduced by allopurinol, and that the adding back of uric acid in allopurinol-treated cells can reinduce the mitochondrial oxidative stress [62].

Limitations to the Fructose-Uric Acid Hypothesis for Metabolic Syndrome and Diabetes

There are 2 major limitations to the uric acid and metabolic syndrome hypothesis. The first main concern is that Mendelian randomization studies have reported that genetic polymorphisms that can predict hyperuricemia and gout do not predict the development of diabetes [113–115]. Since Mendelian randomization can remove confounding effects of environment, these studies would suggest that serum uric acid may not have a causal role in diabetes. However, this could reflect the possibility that the polymorphisms may not correlate with intracellular uric acid levels, which is where the uric acid is expected to have its biological action, and it also does not take into account the interacting effects of diet and/or environment. The second concern is the lack of well-powered, placebo-controlled randomized clinical trials to determine the benefit of lowering uric acid on prediabetes and preventing the development of diabetes.

Conclusions

In summary, it has long been known that subjects with chronic hyperuricemia and/or gout are found to be associated with obesity, metabolic syndrome, and diabetes. Indeed, hyperuricemia is an independent risk factor for the development of type 2 diabetes. Experimental studies also suggest a role for uric acid in mediating both fructose-dependent and fructose-independent models of metabolic syndrome. The mechanism is likely mediated by mitochondrial oxidative stress that may alter AKT phosphorylation and also effects on endothelial function. Early clinical trials also show the potential benefit of lowering serum uric acid on blood pressure and insulin resistance. Larger clinical trials are now needed to assess the potential benefit of lowering uric acid on the incidence of type 2 diabetes.

References

1 Lancereaux E: Le Diabete Maigre et le Diabete Gras. L' Union Mid 1880.

2 Duckworth D: A Treatise on Gout. London, C. Griffin & Co., 1889.

3 Haig A: Uric Acid as a Factor in the Causation of Disease. A Contribution to the Pathology of High Arterial Tension, Headache, Epilepsy, Mental Depression, Gout, Rheumatism, Diabetes, Bright's Disease, and Other Disorders. London, J & A Churchill, 1892.

4 Kylin E: [Studies of the hypertension-hyperglycemia-hyperuricemia syndrome] Studien über das Hypertonie-Hyperglykamie-Hyperurikamiesyndrome. Zentralblatt fur Innere Medizin 1923;44:105–127.
5 McKechnie JK: Gout, Hyperuricaemia and Carbohydrate Metabolism. S Afr Med J 1964; 38:182–185.
6 Prior IA, Rose BS, Davidson F: Metabolic maladies in New Zealand maoris. Br Med J 1964;1:1065–1069.
7 Healey LA, Caner JE, Basset DR, Decker JL: Serum uric acid and obesity in Hawaiians. JAMA 1966;196:364–365.
8 Prior IA, Rose BS, Harvey HP, Davidson F: Hyperuricaemia, gout, and diabetic abnormality in Polynesian people. Lancet 1966;1: 333–338.
9 Buchanan KD: Diabetes mellitus and gout. Semin Arthritis Rheum 1972;2:157–163.
10 Herman JB, Medalie JH, Goldbourt U: Diabetes, prediabetes and uricaemia. Diabetologia 1976;12:47–52.
11 Reaven GM: Banting Lecture 1988. Role of insulin resistance in human disease. 1988. Nutrition 1997;13:65; discussion 64, 66.
12 Facchini F, Chen YD, Hollenbeck CB, Reaven GM: Relationship between resistance to insulin-mediated glucose uptake, urinary uric acid clearance, and plasma uric acid concentration. JAMA 1991;266:3008–3011.
13 Quinones GA, Natali A, Baldi S, Frascerra S, Sanna G, Ciociaro D, Ferrannini E: Effect of insulin on uric acid excretion in humans. Am J Physiol 1995;268:E1–E5.
14 Meigs JB: Invited commentary: insulin resistance syndrome? Syndrome X? Multiple metabolic syndrome? A syndrome at all? Factor analysis reveals patterns in the fabric of correlated metabolic risk factors. Am J Epidemiol 2000;152:908–911; discussion 912.
15 Kahn R, Buse J, Ferrannini E, Stern M: The metabolic syndrome: time for a critical appraisal: joint statement from the American Diabetes Association and the European Association for the Study of Diabetes. Diabetes Care 2005;28:2289–2304.
16 Grundy SM: Does the metabolic syndrome exist? Diabetes Care 2006;29:1689–1692; discussion 1693–1686.
17 Brietzke SA: Controversy in diagnosis and management of the metabolic syndrome. Med Clin North Am 2007;91:1041–1061, vii–viii.
18 Reaven GM: The metabolic syndrome: time to get off the merry-go-round? J Intern Med 2011;269:127–136.
19 Bairlein F: How to get fat: nutritional mechanisms of seasonal fat accumulation in migratory songbirds. Naturwissenschaften 2002;89: 1–10.
20 Martin SL: Mammalian hibernation: a naturally reversible model for insulin resistance in man? Diab Vasc Dis Res 2008;5:76–81.
21 Lanaspa MA, Epperson LE, Li N, Cicerchi C, Garcia GE, Roncal-Jimenez CA, Trostel J, Jain S, Mant CT, Rivard CJ, Ishimoto T, Shimada M, Sanchez-Lozada LG, Nakagawa T, Jani A, Stenvinkel P, Martin SL, Johnson RJ: Opposing activity changes in AMP deaminase and AMP-activated protein kinase in the hibernating ground squirrel. PLoS One 2015; 10:e0123509.
22 Johnson RJ, Stenvinkel P, Martin SL, Jani A, Sanchez-Lozada LG, Hill JO, Lanaspa MA: Redefining metabolic syndrome as a fat storage condition based on studies of comparative physiology. Obesity (Silver Spring) 2013; 21:659–664.
23 Sahu A: Leptin signaling in the hypothalamus: emphasis on energy homeostasis and leptin resistance. Front Neuroendocrinol 2003;24:225–253.
24 Kim JY, Hickner RC, Cortright RL, Dohm GL, Houmard JA: Lipid oxidation is reduced in obese human skeletal muscle. Am J Physiol Endocrinol Metab 2000;279:E1039–E1044.
25 Cook S, Hugli O, Egli M, Vollenweider P, Burcelin R, Nicod P, Thorens B, Scherrer U: Clustering of cardiovascular risk factors mimicking the human metabolic syndrome X in eNOS null mice. Swiss Med Wkly 2003; 133:360–363.
26 Taveau C, Chollet C, Waeckel L, Desposito D, Bichet DG, Arthus MF, Magnan C, Philippe E, Paradis V, Foufelle F, Hainault I, Enhorning S, Velho G, Roussel R, Bankir L, Melander O, Bouby N: Vasopressin and hydration play a major role in the development of glucose intolerance and hepatic steatosis in obese rats. Diabetologia 2015;58:1081–1090.
27 Johnson RJ, Stenvinkel P, Jensen T, Lanaspa MA, Roncal C, Song Z, Bankir L, Sanchez-Lozada LG: Metabolic and kidney diseases in the setting of climate change, water shortage, and survival factors. J Am Soc Nephrol 2016; 27:2247–2256.

28 Malik VS, Pan A, Willett WC, Hu FB: Sugar-sweetened beverages and weight gain in children and adults: a systematic review and meta-analysis. Am J Clin Nutr 2013;98: 1084–1102.

29 Malik VS, Popkin BM, Bray GA, Despres JP, Willett WC, Hu FB: Sugar-sweetened beverages and risk of metabolic syndrome and type 2 diabetes: a meta-analysis. Diabetes Care 2010;33:2477–2483.

30 Nakagawa T, Hu H, Zharikov S, Tuttle KR, Short RA, Glushakova O, Ouyang X, Feig DI, Block ER, Herrera-Acosta J, Patel JM, Johnson RJ: A causal role for uric acid in fructose-induced metabolic syndrome. Am J Physiol Renal Physiol 2006;290:F625–F631.

31 Reungjui S, Pratipanawatr T, Johnson RJ, Nakagawa T: Do thiazides worsen metabolic syndrome and renal disease? The pivotal roles for hyperuricemia and hypokalemia. Curr Opin Nephrol Hypertens 2008;17:470–476.

32 Gersch MS, Mu W, Cirillo P, Reungjui S, Zhang L, Roncal C, Sautin YY, Johnson RJ, Nakagawa T: Fructose, but not dextrose, accelerates the progression of chronic kidney disease. Am J Physiol Renal Physiol 2007; 293:F1256–F1261.

33 Cox CL, Stanhope KL, Schwarz JM, Graham JL, Hatcher B, Griffen SC, Bremer AA, Berglund L, McGahan JP, Havel PJ, Keim NL: Consumption of fructose-sweetened beverages for 10 weeks reduces net fat oxidation and energy expenditure in overweight/obese men and women. Eur J Clin Nutr 2012;66: 201–208.

34 Stanhope KL, Griffen SC, Keim NL, Ai M, Otokozawa S, Nakajima K, Schaefer E, Havel PJ: Consumption of fructose-, but not glucose-sweetened beverages produces an atherogenic lipid profile in overweight/obese men and women. Diabetes 2007;56(suppl 1):A16.

35 Stanhope KL, Schwarz JM, Keim NL, Griffen SC, Bremer AA, Graham JL, Hatcher B, Cox CL, Dyachenko A, Zhang W, McGahan JP, Seibert A, Krauss RM, Chiu S, Schaefer EJ, Ai M, Otokozawa S, Nakajima K, Nakano T, Beysen C, Hellerstein MK, Berglund L, Havel PJ: Consuming fructose-sweetened, not glucose-sweetened, beverages increases visceral adiposity and lipids and decreases insulin sensitivity in overweight/obese humans. J Clin Invest 2009;119:1322–1334.

36 Lanaspa MA, Ishimoto T, Li N, Cicerchi C, Orlicky DJ, Ruzycki P, Rivard C, Inaba S, Roncal-Jimenez CA, Bales ES, Diggle CP, Asipu A, Petrash JM, Kosugi T, Maruyama S, Sanchez-Lozada LG, McManaman JL, Bonthron DT, Sautin YY, Johnson RJ: Endogenous fructose production and metabolism in the liver contributes to the development of metabolic syndrome. Nat Commun 2013;4: 2434.

37 Fox IH, Kelley WN: Studies on the mechanism of fructose-induced hyperuricemia in man. Metabolism 1972;21:713–721.

38 Raivio KO, Becker A, Meyer LJ, Greene ML, Nuki G, Seegmiller JE: Stimulation of human purine synthesis de novo by fructose infusion. Metabolism 1975;24:861–869.

39 Diggle CP, Shires M, Leitch D, Brooke D, Carr IM, Markham AF, Hayward BE, Asipu A, Bonthron DT: Ketohexokinase: expression and localization of the principal fructose-metabolizing enzyme. J Histochem Cytochem 2009;57:763–774.

40 Oppelt SA, Zhang W, Tolan DR: Specific regions of the brain are capable of fructose metabolism. Brain Res 2017;1657:312–322.

41 Song Z, Roncal-Jimenez CA, Lanaspa-Garcia MA, Oppelt SA, Kuwabara M, Jensen T, Milagres T, Andres-Hernando A, Ishimoto T, Garcia GE, Johnson G, MacLean PS, Sanchez-Lozada LG, Tolan DR, Johnson RJ: Role of fructose and fructokinase in acute dehydration-induced vasopressin gene expression and secretion in mice. J Neurophysiol 2017; 117:646–654.

42 Woods HF, Eggleston LV, Krebs HA: The cause of hepatic accumulation of fructose 1-phosphate on fructose loading. Biochem J 1970;119:501–510.

43 van den Berghe G, Bronfman M, Vanneste R, Hers HG: The mechanism of adenosine triphosphate depletion in the liver after a load of fructose. A kinetic study of liver adenylate deaminase. Biochem J 1977;162:601–609.

44 Lanaspa MA, Cicerchi C, Garcia G, Li N, Roncal-Jimenez CA, Rivard CJ, Hunter B, Andres-Hernando A, Ishimoto T, Sanchez-Lozada LG, Thomas J, Hodges RS, Mant CT, Johnson RJ: Counteracting roles of AMP deaminase and AMP kinase in the development of fatty liver. PLoS One 2012;7:e48801.

45 Cicerchi C, Li N, Kratzer J, Garcia G, Roncal-Jimenez CA, Tanabe K, Hunter B, Rivard CJ, Sautin YY, Gaucher EA, Johnson RJ, Lanaspa MA: Uric acid-dependent inhibition of AMP kinase induces hepatic glucose production in diabetes and starvation: evolutionary implications of the uricase loss in hominids. FASEB J 2014;28:3339–3350.
46 Zhang Y, Hong Q, Huang Z, Xue P, Lv Y, Fu B, Chen X, Wu D: ALDR enhanced endothelial injury in hyperuricemia screened using SILAC. Cell Physiol Biochem 2014;33:479–490.
47 Lanaspa MA, Sanchez-Lozada LG, Cicerchi C, Li N, Roncal-Jimenez CA, Ishimoto T, Le M, Garcia GE, Thomas JB, Rivard CJ, Andres-Hernando A, Hunter B, Schreiner G, Rodriguez-Iturbe B, Sautin YY, Johnson RJ: Uric acid stimulates fructokinase and accelerates fructose metabolism in the development of fatty liver. PLoS One 2012;7:e47948.
48 Radi R, Tan S, Prodanov E, Evans RA, Parks DA: Inhibition of xanthine oxidase by uric acid and its influence on superoxide radical production. Biochim Biophys Acta 1992; 1122:178–182.
49 Tan S, Radi R, Gaudier F, Evans RA, Rivera A, Kirk KA, Parks DA: Physiologic levels of uric acid inhibit xanthine oxidase in human plasma. Pediatr Res 1993;34:303–307.
50 Cirillo P, Gersch MS, Mu W, Scherer PM, Kim KM, Gesualdo L, Henderson GN, Johnson RJ, Sautin YY: Ketohexokinase-dependent metabolism of fructose induces proinflammatory mediators in proximal tubular cells. J Am Soc Nephrol 2009;20:545–553.
51 Le MT, Frye RF, Rivard CJ, Cheng J, McFann KK, Segal MS, Johnson RJ, Johnson JA: Effects of high-fructose corn syrup and sucrose on the pharmacokinetics of fructose and acute metabolic and hemodynamic responses in healthy subjects. Metabolism 2012;61:641–651.
52 Stirpe F, Della Corte E, Bonetti E, Abbondanza A, Abbati A, De Stefano F: Fructose-induced hyperuricaemia. Lancet 1970;2:1310–1311.
53 Cox CL, Stanhope KL, Schwarz JM, Graham JL, Hatcher B, Griffen SC, Bremer AA, Berglund L, McGahan JP, Keim NL, Havel PJ: Consumption of fructose- but not glucose-sweetened beverages for 10 weeks increases circulating concentrations of uric acid, retinol binding protein-4, and gamma-glutamyl transferase activity in overweight/obese humans. Nutr Metab (Lond) 2012;9:68.
54 Choi JW, Ford ES, Gao X, Choi HK: Sugar-sweetened soft drinks, diet soft drinks, and serum uric acid level: the third national health and nutrition examination survey. Arthritis Rheum 2007;59:109–116.
55 Kanellis J, Watanabe S, Li JH, Kang DH, Li P, Nakagawa T, Wamsley A, Sheikh-Hamad D, Lan HY, Feng L, Johnson RJ: Uric acid stimulates monocyte chemoattractant protein-1 production in vascular smooth muscle cells via mitogen-activated protein kinase and cyclooxygenase-2. Hypertension 2003;41:1287–1293.
56 Kang DH, Park SK, Lee IK, Johnson RJ: Uric acid-induced C-reactive protein expression: implication on cell proliferation and nitric oxide production of human vascular cells. J Am Soc Nephrol 2005;16:3553–3562.
57 Corry DB, Eslami P, Yamamoto K, Nyby MD, Makino H, Tuck ML: Uric acid stimulates vascular smooth muscle cell proliferation and oxidative stress via the vascular renin-angiotensin system. J Hypertens 2008;26: 269–275.
58 Yu MA, Sanchez-Lozada LG, Johnson RJ, Kang DH: Oxidative stress with an activation of the renin-angiotensin system in human vascular endothelial cells as a novel mechanism of uric acid-induced endothelial dysfunction. J Hypertens 2010;28:1234–1242.
59 Khosla UM, Zharikov S, Finch JL, Nakagawa T, Roncal C, Mu W, Krotova K, Block ER, Prabhakar S, Johnson RJ: Hyperuricemia induces endothelial dysfunction. Kidney Int 2005;67:1739–1742.
60 Sanchez-Lozada LG, Tapia E, Bautista-Garcia P, Soto V, Avila-Casado C, Vega-Campos IP, Nakagawa T, Zhao L, Franco M, Johnson RJ: Effects of febuxostat on metabolic and renal alterations in rats with fructose-induced metabolic syndrome. Am J Physiol Renal Physiol 2008;294:F710–F718.

61 Baldwin W, McRae S, Marek G, Wymer D, Pannu V, Baylis C, Johnson RJ, Sautin YY: Hyperuricemia as a mediator of the proinflammatory endocrine imbalance in the adipose tissue in a murine model of the metabolic syndrome. Diabetes 2011;60:1258–1269.
62 Lanaspa MA, Sanchez-Lozada LG, Choi YJ, Cicerchi C, Kanbay M, Roncal-Jimenez CA, Ishimoto T, Li N, Marek G, Duranay M, Schreiner G, Rodriguez-Iturbe B, Nakagawa T, Kang DH, Sautin YY, Johnson RJ: Uric acid induces hepatic steatosis by generation of mitochondrial oxidative stress: potential role in fructose-dependent and -independent fatty liver. J Biol Chem 2012;287:40732–40744.
63 Choi HK, Ford ES: Prevalence of the metabolic syndrome in individuals with hyperuricemia. Am J Med 2007;120:442–447.
64 Choi HK, Ford ES, Li C, Curhan G: Prevalence of the metabolic syndrome in patients with gout: the Third National Health and Nutrition Examination Survey. Arthritis Rheum 2007;57:109–115.
65 Kuwabara M, Niwa K, Hisatome I, Nakagawa T, Roncal-Jimenez CA, Andres-Hernando A, Bjornstad P, Jensen T, Sato Y, Milagres T, Garcia G, Ohno M, Lanaspa MA, Johnson RJ: Asymptomatic hyperuricemia without comorbidities predicts cardiometabolic diseases: five-year Japanese cohort study. Hypertension 2017;69:1036–1044.
66 Dehghan A, van Hoek M, Sijbrands EJ, Hofman A, Witteman JC: High serum uric acid as a novel risk factor for type 2 diabetes. Diabetes Care 2008;31:361–362.
67 Kodama S, Saito K, Yachi Y, Asumi M, Sugawara A, Totsuka K, Saito A, Sone H: Association between serum uric acid and development of type 2 diabetes. Diabetes Care 2009; 32:1737–1742.
68 Balkau B, King H, Zimmet P, Raper LR: Factors associated with the development of diabetes in the Micronesian population of Nauru. Am J Epidemiol 1985;122:594–605.
69 Bhole V, Choi JW, Kim SW, de Vera M, Choi H: Serum uric acid levels and the risk of type 2 diabetes: a prospective study. Am J Med 2010;123:957–961.
70 Boyko EJ, de Courten M, Zimmet PZ, Chitson P, Tuomilehto J, Alberti KG: Features of the metabolic syndrome predict higher risk of diabetes and impaired glucose tolerance: a prospective study in Mauritius. Diabetes Care 2000;23:1242–1248.
71 Chien KL, Chen MF, Hsu HC, Chang WT, Su TC, Lee YT, Hu FB: Plasma uric acid and the risk of type 2 diabetes in a Chinese community. Clin Chem 2008;54:310–316.
72 Kramer CK, von Muhlen D, Jassal SK, Barrett-Connor E: Serum uric acid levels improve prediction of incident type 2 diabetes in individuals with impaired fasting glucose: the Rancho Bernardo Study. Diabetes Care 2009;32:1272–1273.
73 Krishnan E, Pandya BJ, Chung L, Hariri A, Dabbous O: Hyperuricemia in young adults and risk of insulin resistance, prediabetes, and diabetes: a 15-year follow-up study. Am J Epidemiol 2012;176:108–116.
74 Lv Q, Meng XF, He FF, Chen S, Su H, Xiong J, Gao P, Tian XJ, Liu JS, Zhu ZH, Huang K, Zhang C: High serum uric acid and increased risk of type 2 diabetes: a systemic review and meta-analysis of prospective cohort studies. PLoS One 2013;8:e56864.
75 Nan H, Qiao Q, Soderberg S, Pitkaniemi J, Zimmet P, Shaw J, Alberti G, Uusitalo U, Pauvaday V, Chitson P, Tuomilehto J: Serum uric acid and incident diabetes in Mauritian Indian and Creole populations. Diabetes Res Clin Pract 2008;80:321–327.
76 Ohlson LO, Larsson B, Bjorntorp P, Eriksson H, Svardsudd K, Welin L, Tibblin G, Wilhelmsen L: Risk factors for type 2 (non-insulin-dependent) diabetes mellitus. Thirteen and one-half years of follow-up of the participants in a study of Swedish men born in 1913. Diabetologia 1988;31:798–805.
77 Perry IJ, Wannamethee SG, Walker MK, Thomson AG, Whincup PH, Shaper AG: Prospective study of risk factors for development of non-insulin dependent diabetes in middle aged British men. BMJ 1995;310:560–564.
78 Masuo K, Kawaguchi H, Mikami H, Ogihara T, Tuck ML: Serum uric acid and plasma norepinephrine concentrations predict subsequent weight gain and blood pressure elevation. Hypertension 2003;42:474–480.
79 Sirota JC, McFann K, Targher G, Johnson RJ, Chonchol M, Jalal DI: Elevated serum uric acid levels are associated with non-alcoholic fatty liver disease independently of metabolic syndrome features in the United States: Liver ultrasound data from the National Health and Nutrition Examination Survey. Metabolism 2013;62:392–399.

80 Lee JW, Cho YK, Ryan M, Kim H, Lee SW, Chang E, Joo KJ, Kim JT, Kim BS, Sung KC: Serum uric acid as a predictor for the development of nonalcoholic fatty liver disease in apparently healthy subjects: a 5-year retrospective cohort study. Gut Liver 2010;4:378–383.
81 Ryu S, Chang Y, Kim SG, Cho J, Guallar E: Serum uric acid levels predict incident nonalcoholic fatty liver disease in healthy Korean men. Metabolism 2011;60:860–866.
82 Xu C, Yu C, Xu L, Miao M, Li Y: High serum uric acid increases the risk for nonalcoholic fatty liver disease: a prospective observational study. PLoS One 2010;5:e11578.
83 Yamada T, Suzuki S, Fukatsu M, Wada T, Yoshida T, Joh T: Elevated serum uric acid is an independent risk factor for nonalcoholic fatty liver disease in Japanese undergoing a health checkup. Acta Gastroenterol Belg 2010;73:12–17.
84 Grayson PC, Kim SY, LaValley M, Choi HK: Hyperuricemia and incident hypertension: a systematic review and meta-analysis. Arthritis Care Res (Hoboken) 2011;63:102–110.
85 Feig DI, Madero M, Jalal DI, Sanchez-Lozada LG, Johnson RJ: Uric acid and the origins of hypertension. J Pediatr 2013;162:896–902.
86 Takir M, Kostek O, Ozkok A, Elcioglu OC, Bakan A, Erek A, Mutlu HH, Telci O, Semerci A, Odabas AR, Afsar B, Smits G, ALanaspa M, Sharma S, Johnson RJ, Kanbay M: Lowering uric acid with allopurinol improves insulin resistance and systemic inflammation in asymptomatic hyperuricemia. J Investig Med 2015;63:924–929.
87 Liu P, Chen Y, Wang B, Zhang F, Wang D, Wang Y: Allopurinol treatment improves renal function in patients with type 2 diabetes and asymptomatic hyperuricemia: 3-year randomized parallel-controlled study. Clin Endocrinol (Oxf) 2015;83:475–482.
88 Meng J, Li Y, Yuan X, Lu Y: Effects of febuxostat on insulin resistance and expression of high-sensitivity C-reactive protein in patients with primary gout. Rheumatol Int 2017;37:299–303.
89 Ogino K, Kato M, Furuse Y, Kinugasa Y, Ishida K, Osaki S, Kinugawa T, Igawa O, Hisatome I, Shigemasa C, Anker SD, Doehner W: Uric acid-lowering treatment with benzbromarone in patients with heart failure: a double-blind placebo-controlled crossover preliminary study. Circ Heart Fail 2010;3:73–81.
90 Sedhom SS, Badary OA, Salama SH, Mokhles MA: Assessment of the therapeutic effect of allopurinol on patients with non-alcoholic fatty liver disease associated with hyperuricemia by cytokeratin 18. J Gastrointest Dig Syst 6:http://dx.doi.org/10.4172/2161-4069X.C4171.4044 (Abstract), 2016.
91 Perez-Pozo SE, Schold J, Nakagawa T, Sanchez-Lozada LG, Johnson RJ, Lillo JL: Excessive fructose intake induces the features of metabolic syndrome in healthy adult men: role of uric acid in the hypertensive response. Int J Obes (Lond) 2010;34:454–461.
92 Soletsky B, Feig DI: Uric acid reduction rectifies prehypertension in obese adolescents. Hypertension 2012;60:1148–1156.
93 Madero M, Rodriguez Castellanos FE, Jalal D, Villalobos-Martin M, Salazar J, Vazquez-Rangel A, Johnson RJ, Sanchez-Lozada LG: A pilot study on the impact of a low fructose diet and allopurinol on clinic blood pressure among overweight and prehypertensive subjects: a randomized placebo controlled trial. J Am Soc Hypertens 2015;9:837–844.
94 Sanchez-Lozada LG, Soto V, Tapia E, Avila-Casado C, Sautin YY, Nakagawa T, Franco M, Rodriguez-Iturbe B, Johnson RJ: Role of oxidative stress in the renal abnormalities induced by experimental hyperuricemia. Am J Physiol Renal Physiol 2008;295:F1134–F1141.
95 Sanchez-Lozada LG, Tapia E, Lopez-Molina R, Nepomuceno T, Soto V, Avila-Casado C, Nakagawa T, Johnson RJ, Herrera-Acosta J, Franco M: Effects of acute and chronic L-arginine treatment in experimental hyperuricemia. Am J Physiol Renal Physiol 2007;292:F1238–F1244.
96 Mazzali M, Hughes J, Kim YG, Jefferson JA, Kang DH, Gordon KL, Lan HY, Kivlighn S, Johnson RJ: Elevated uric acid increases blood pressure in the rat by a novel crystal-independent mechanism. Hypertension 2001;38:1101–1106.
97 Mazzali M, Kanellis J, Han L, Feng L, Xia YY, Chen Q, Kang DH, Gordon KL, Watanabe S, Nakagawa T, Lan HY, Johnson RJ: Hyperuricemia induces a primary renal arteriolopathy in rats by a blood pressure-independent mechanism. Am J Physiol Renal Physiol 2002;282:F991–F997.

98 Sautin YY, Nakagawa T, Zharikov S, Johnson RJ: Adverse effects of the classic antioxidant uric acid in adipocytes: NADPH oxidase-mediated oxidative/nitrosative stress. Am J Physiol Cell Physiol 2007;293:C584–C596.
99 Choi YJ, Shin HS, Choi HS, Park JW, Jo I, Oh ES, Lee KY, Lee BH, Johnson RJ, Kang DH: Uric acid induces fat accumulation via generation of endoplasmic reticulum stress and SREBP-1c activation in hepatocytes. Lab Invest 2014;94:1114–1125.
100 Ames BN, Cathcart R, Schwiers E, Hochstein P: Uric acid provides an antioxidant defense in humans against oxidant- and radical-caused aging and cancer: a hypothesis. Proc Natl Acad Sci U S A 1981;78: 6858–6862.
101 Robinson KM, Morre JT, Beckman JS: Triuret: a novel product of peroxynitrite-mediated oxidation of urate. Arch Biochem Biophys 2004;423:213–217.
102 Gersch C, Palii SP, Imaram W, Kim KM, Karumanchi SA, Angerhofer A, Johnson RJ, Henderson GN: Reactions of peroxynitrite with uric acid: formation of reactive intermediates, alkylated products and triuret, and in vivo production of triuret under conditions of oxidative stress. Nucleosides Nucleotides Nucleic Acids 2009;28:118–149.
103 Imaram W, Gersch C, Kim KM, Johnson RJ, Henderson GN, Angerhofer A: Radicals in the reaction between peroxynitrite and uric acid identified by electron spin resonance spectroscopy and liquid chromatography mass spectrometry. Free Radic Biol Med 2010;49:275–281.
104 Carvalho LA, Truzzi DR, Fallani TS, Alves SV, Toledo JC Jr, Augusto O, Netto LES, Meotti FC: Urate hydroperoxide oxidizes human peroxiredoxin 1 and peroxiredoxin 2. J Biol Chem 2017;292:8705–8715.
105 Patricio ES, Prado FM, da Silva RP, Carvalho LA, Prates MV, Dadamos T, Bertotti M, Di Mascio P, Kettle AJ, Meotti FC: Chemical characterization of urate hydroperoxide, a pro-oxidant intermediate generated by urate oxidation in inflammatory and photoinduced processes. Chem Res Toxicol 2015;28:1556–1566.
106 Verzola D, Ratto E, Villaggio B, Parodi EL, Pontremoli R, Garibotto G, Viazzi F: Uric acid promotes apoptosis in human proximal tubule cells by oxidative stress and the activation of NADPH oxidase NOX 4. PLoS One 2014;9:e115210.
107 Block K, Gorin Y, Abboud HE: Subcellular localization of Nox4 and regulation in diabetes. Proc Natl Acad Sci U S A 2009;106: 14385–14390.
108 Ago T, Kuroda J, Pain J, Fu C, Li H, Sadoshima J: Upregulation of Nox4 by hypertrophic stimuli promotes apoptosis and mitochondrial dysfunction in cardiac myocytes. Circ Res 2010;106:1253–1264.
109 Sanchez-Lozada LG, Lanaspa MA, Cristobal-Garcia M, Garcia-Arroyo F, Soto V, Cruz-Robles D, Nakagawa T, Yu MA, Kang DH, Johnson RJ: Uric acid-induced endothelial dysfunction is associated with mitochondrial alterations and decreased intracellular ATP concentrations. Nephron Exp Nephrol 2012;121:e71–e78.
110 Vieceli Dalla Sega F, Zambonin L, Fiorentini D, Rizzo B, Caliceti C, Landi L, Hrelia S, Prata C: Specific aquaporins facilitate Nox-produced hydrogen peroxide transport through plasma membrane in leukaemia cells. Biochim Biophys Acta 2014;1843:806–814.
111 Bienert GP, Schjoerring JK, Jahn TP: Membrane transport of hydrogen peroxide. Biochim Biophys Acta 2006;1758:994–1003.
112 Wani R, Qian J, Yin L, Bechtold E, King SB, Poole LB, Paek E, Tsang AW, Furdui CM: Isoform-specific regulation of Akt by PDGF-induced reactive oxygen species. Proc Natl Acad Sci U S A 2011;108:10550–10555.
113 Pfister R, Barnes D, Luben R, Forouhi NG, Bochud M, Khaw KT, Wareham NJ, Langenberg C: No evidence for a causal link between uric acid and type 2 diabetes: a Mendelian randomisation approach. Diabetologia 2011;54:2561–2569.

114 Yang Q, Kottgen A, Dehghan A, Smith AV, Glazer NL, Chen MH, Chasman DI, Aspelund T, Eiriksdottir G, Harris TB, Launer L, Nalls M, Hernandez D, Arking DE, Boerwinkle E, Grove ML, Li M, Linda Kao WH, Chonchol M, Haritunians T, Li G, Lumley T, Psaty BM, Shlipak M, Hwang SJ, Larson MG, O'Donnell CJ, Upadhyay A, van Duijn CM, Hofman A, Rivadeneira F, Stricker B, Uitterlinden AG, Pare G, Parker AN, Ridker PM, Siscovick DS, Gudnason V, Witteman JC, Fox CS, Coresh J: Multiple genetic loci influence serum urate levels and their relationship with gout and cardiovascular disease risk factors. Circ Cardiovasc Genet 2010;3:523–530.

115 Dehghan A, Kottgen A, Yang Q, Hwang SJ, Kao WL, Rivadeneira F, Boerwinkle E, Levy D, Hofman A, Astor BC, Benjamin EJ, van Duijn CM, Witteman JC, Coresh J, Fox CS: Association of three genetic loci with uric acid concentration and risk of gout: a genome-wide association study. Lancet 2008; 372:1953–1961.

Richard J. Johnson, MD
Division of Renal Diseases and Hypertension
12700 East 19th Ave
Aurora, CO 80045 (USA)
E-Mail Richard.Johnson@ucdenver.edu

Treviño-Becerra A, Iseki K (eds): Uric Acid in Chronic Kidney Disease.
Contrib Nephrol. Basel, Karger, 2018, vol 192, pp 103–109 (DOI: 10.1159/000484284)

Uric Acid and Diabetic Nephropathy Risk

Michael Mauer[a] · Alessandro Doria[b]

[a]Department of Pediatrics and Medicine, University of Minnesota School of Medicine, Minneapolis, MN, and [b]Research Division, Joslin Diabetes Center, Department of Medicine, Harvard School of Medicine, Boston, MA, USA

Abstract

Background: Diabetic nephropathy (DN) is the leading cause of end-stage renal disease (ESRD) in the western world. Current treatment methods, with better control of glycemia and blood pressure, including renin-angiotensin system blockade (RASB), appear to have slowed the DN progression rate but have not substantially decreased the annual incidence of new DN ESRD cases. Thus, new treatment targets are needed. ***Summary:*** Higher levels of serum uric acid (UA) are associated with increased risk of the clinical manifestations of DN in persons with types 1 and 2 diabetes. Also, UA is a strong predictor of DN progression. Two small, short-term, proof-of-concept clinical trials in which a minority of the patients had diabetes suggested that reduction of UA with allopurinol could decrease the rate of glomerular filtration rate (GFR) loss in persons with chronic kidney disease (CKD). However, a definitive trial to check whether UA reduction can benefit DN progression has not been conducted as yet. Preventing Early Renal Loss in Diabetes (PERL) is an ongoing trial in persons with type 1 diabetes and early to moderate GFR reduction. This 3-year randomized placebo controlled trial in 530 subjects is to check whether UA reduction with allopurinol can slow the rate of GFR decline as determined by the plasma disappearance of iohexol. ***Key Message:*** If the results of the PERL trial are positive, initiation of UA reduction treatment while GFR is relatively well preserved could delay ESRD in DN by 8–10 years, that is, considerably longer than the period that has been demonstrated for RASB. This could have important implications for the treatment of DN in particular and of CKD in general.

Introduction

Diabetic nephropathy (DN) is the most common cause of end-stage renal disease (ESRD) in the western world, representing ~46% of all new ESRD cases in the United States [1]. In spite of all the improvements achieved to control glycemia [2] and blood pressure and despite the use of renin angiotensin system blocking (RASB) drugs [3], the USA annual incidence of diabetes related ESRD continues to rise [1], and the full impact of the recent marked increases in obesity and diabetes incidence is yet to be felt for this long-term diabetes complication. This is particularly worrisome, given that nearly half of all patients with diabetes fail to maintain HbA1c values below 7% [4]. Importantly, the beneficial impact of RASB in patients with diabetes and established DN was only seen in those with estimated glomerular filtration rate (eGFRs) <60 mL/min/1.73 m^2 [3] and the extension of renal survival in those cases was generally less than 2 years. Thus, new treatment methods are needed, especially ones that, in addition to being effective in slowing or preventing DN, are safe, relatively inexpensive, and therefore reasonable to institute at earlier stages of the disease. Allopurinol, a xanthine oxidase inhibitor, which lowers uric acid (UA), is such a drug and this review examines the clinical evidence linking higher levels of serum UA (SUA) with DN risk and progression and argues for definitive trials to test the hypothesis that SUA reduction would benefit persons with diabetes at increased risk of DN.

Serum UA as a Predictor of the Development of DN

The Steno cohort study included all newly diagnosed type 1 diabetic (T1D) patients consecutively admitted to the Steno Diabetes Center between September 1979 and August 1984. This inception cohort had baseline SUA measured 3 years after the onset of diabetes, that is, before any patient developed microalbuminuria (MA) [5] and was followed up for a median of 18.1 (interquartile range 1.0–21.8) years. Patients in the highest quartile of SUA values (>4.2 mg/dL) had a 25% risk of developing macroalbuminuria during follow-up as compared to a 10% risk in the lower 3 SUA quartiles (p = 0.006). Adjustment for baseline body mass index (BMI), glycemia, albumin excretion rate, serum creatinine (SCr), serum cholesterol, and mean arterial blood pressure did not significantly change the results (adjusted HR 2.93 [1.25–6.86] per 1.7 mg/dL (100 μmol/L) increase in SUA; p = 0.013) [5]. However, SUA was not a predictor of MA or measured GFR loss.

Pacilli et al. [6] studied the epidemiology of DN in 20,464 adult patients with T1D in Italy, 11,162 of whom had information available on SUA. SUA was strongly associated with DN (OR 1.56; 95% CI 1.49–1.63; $p < 0.001$), low eGFR (<60 mL/min/1.73 m^2, OR 2.31; 95% CI 2.17–2.47; $p < 0.001$), and albuminuria (OR 1.30; 95% CI 1.25–1.36; $p < 0.001$) for each 1 mg/dL increase of SUA levels.

Zoppini et al. [7] followed 1,449 T2D patients with eGFR >60 mL/min/1.73 m^2 and no overt proteinuria for the incidence of new onset chronic kidney disease (CKD) defined as overt proteinuria or eGFR <60 mL/min/1.73 m^2. Hyperuricemia in this study was defined as SUA ≥7.0 mg/dL in men and ≥6.5 mg/dL in women. During 5-years of follow-up, the CKD cumulative incidence was 29.5% in patients with hyperuricemia vs. 11.4% in those without ($p = 0.001$). In univariate logistic regression analysis, hyperuricemia was associated with a 2.5-fold increase in CKD risk (OR 2.55 [95% CI 1.71–3.85], $p = 0.001$) [7]. After adjusting for age, sex, BMI, smoking, T2D duration, BP, BP treatment, insulin therapy, HbA1c, eGFR, and albuminuria, hyperuricemia remained associated with increased CKD risk (adjusted OR 2.10 [1.16–3.76], $p = 0.01$). This corresponded to a 21% increase in CKD risk for each 1-SD increment in SUA [7].

Jalal et al. [8] studied 455 normoalbuminuric T1D patients to determine whether baseline SUA predicted the development of micro- or macroalbuminuria during a 6-year follow-up. In the 324 patients (71%) who completed the study and had available data on change in albuminuria status [8], baseline SUA was significantly higher in the 25 subjects who had progressed to micro- or macroalbuminuria vs. the 299 whose status was unchanged ($p = 0.02$). The receiver operating characteristic curve for SUA, HbA_{1c}, and urinary albumin/creatinine ratio (ACR) provided a c-statistic of 0.82 [8]. When covariates such as sex, age, T1D duration, RASB treatment, waist circumference, waist/hip ratio, BMI, BP, HbA1c, pre-albuminuria, SCr, cystatin C, HDL cholesterol, and triglycerides were included in the regression model, baseline SUA yielded an adjusted OR of 1.8 ($p = 0.005$), that is, similar to the ORs for ACR and HbA1c [8].

Ahola et al. [9], reporting on behalf of the FinnDiane Study Group, found a significant association between increasing SUA levels and worsening DN status in 2,720 patients with T1D. However, in a Mendelian randomization analysis using 25 known genetic predictors of SUA levels, no evidence of causality was found for the relationship between SUA levels and DN progression. These findings suggest that the metabolic phenotype of which SUA is expression (e.g., xanthine oxidase hyperactivity), rather than SUA itself, may be responsible for the increased risk of DN progression associated with increased SUA levels.

Serum UA as a Predictor of DN Progression

In the T1D Joslin Kidney Study, patients with MA ($n = 355$) and baseline eGFR >60 mL/min/1.73 m^2 were evaluated for the outcome of a rate of GFR loss >3.3%/year (above the 95th %tile of normal) during a 6-year follow-up. These patients showed a continuously increasing risk for rapid eGFR decline with increasing SUA levels ranging from <3.0 to >6.0 mg/dL ($p = 0.0002$) [10]. SUA also predicted the risk of developing CKD 3 ($p = 0.0005$) [10] but did not predict ACR progression in these subjects. At baseline, patients with GFR loss >3.3%/year were older and had a longer T1D duration but were similar for $HbA1_C$, insulin dose, BMI, and total or HDL cholesterol [10]. At baseline, patients with rapid GFR loss had significantly lower eGFR, higher ACR, and a greater prevalence of MA. The unadjusted odds ratio for rapid GFR loss was 1.5 (95% CI 1.3–1.9) per 1 mg/d L increment in baseline SUA – an effect that persisted after adjustment for baseline ACR, sex, $HbA1_C$, and eGFR [10].

Hayashino et al. [11] followed 2,518 patients with T2D for 2 years for DN development (transition from normoalbuminuria to micro- or macroalbuminuria) or progression (transition from MA to macroalbuminuria). They assessed the independent correlations between baseline SUA quartiles (means of 3.6, 4.9, 5.8, and 7.3 mg/dL from the 1st–4th quartiles) and outcomes (Cox proportional hazards) adjusted for potential confounders. Baseline SUA quartiles were associated with baseline UACR ($p < 0.001$). As compared to the 2nd quartile, the multivariable-adjusted hazards ratios for progression from MA to macroalbuminuria were 2.17 (95% CI 1.15–4.08; $p = 0.016$) for the 1st quartile, 3.04 (95% CI 1.67–5.53; $p < 0.001$) for the 3rd, and 3.56 (95% CI 1.83–6.93; $p < 0.0011$) for the 4th quartile. There were no significant associations of SUA with progression from NA to MA or with change in eGFR. Given the above information, the association of higher SUA levels with DN progression might have been anticipated, but the increased hazard for lowest SUA quartile was unexpected and unexplained. This group had, numerically, the highest HbA1c level. One possible explanation for this finding could relate to the uricosuric effects of hyperglycemia [12]. This observation needs confirmation and further study.

Chang et al. [13] categorized 2,367 type 2 diabetic patients followed for 3 or more years (mean 4.6) by CKD stage into stable (47.9%), progressing (20.6%), or regressing (31.5%). Multivariate Cox regression analyses were used to identify independent factors associated with change in CKD stage. At baseline, the progression group had the highest (6.9 ± 1.8 mg/dL), and the regression group had the lowest (5.4 ± 1.5 mg/dL) SUA. SUA >6.3 mg/dL was an independent risk factor for CKD progression. In patients with early CKD, almost all at Stage 2, the hazard ratio for progression for higher SUA was 1.54 (95% CI: 1.42–1.68) [13].

Evidence that Reduction in Serum UA Levels Benefits DN Progression

Two small and brief proof-of-concept, placebo-controlled studies with 37% [14] and 25% [15] of the subjects with diabetes suggested that UA reduction with allopurinol could slow CKD progression. More recently, a retrospective 6-month observational study of Febuxostat (a xanthine oxidase inhibitor) suggested, in post hoc analyses, that type 2 diabetic patients achieving an SUA level <6.0 mg/dL benefited by a slight increase in eGFR compared to those not achieving this SUA level [16], but several design weaknesses severely reduced the value of this study.

Losartan can reduce SUA. A post hoc analysis of a 3-year randomized placebo controlled trial of losartan in persons with type 2 diabetes and CKD (RENAAL) showed that participants experiencing an SUA reduction in the first 6 months of the trial had fewer renal events (SCr doubling or ESRD) that those in whom SUA did not decrease [17].

A large 4-year randomized, placebo-controlled primary cardiovascular disease (CVD) trial with the sodium-glucose co-transporter 2 inhibitor empagliflozin demonstrated substantial reductions in CVD endpoints [18]. A post hoc analysis found eGFR preservation and reduced renal events associated with empagliflozin treatment in this study [19]. Among the several hypothesized mechanisms for this outcome was the UA-lowering effect of sodium-glucose co-transporter 2 inhibitors [12, 19].

None of the studies to date are sufficient to adopt SUA reduction as a standard of care for persons with diabetes at increased risk of DN. Nonetheless, taken together, these studies provide the conceptual basis for a large clinical DN trial based on lowering SUA.

The PERL Study: Preventing Early Renal Function Loss in Type 1 Diabetes

Preventing Early Renal Loss in Diabetes (PERL) is a double-blind, placebo-controlled, parallel group, randomized clinical trial being conducted at 16 centers in the United States, Canada, and Denmark [20]. Funded by NIH, and with supplemental funding by JDRF, the study has enrolled 530 persons with type 1 diabetes, eGFR 45–100 ml/min/1.73 m^2, MA/moderate macroalbuminuria OR significant GFR loss (>3 mL/min/1.73 m^2/year) in the previous 3–5 years and serum UA ≥4.5 mg/dL. The primary outcome is the iohexol plasma disappearance measure of GFR (iGFR) at the end of 3 years of intervention and 2 months of drug washout adjusted for the baseline iGFR. Secondary outcomes will include trajectories of eGFR using SCr and or cystatin C, albumin excretion rate, and CVD events. The intervention is SUA reduction with oral allopurinol (200–400 mg once/day, adjusted for eGFR) or placebo (1:1). PERL also follows guidelines and recommendations for RASB in persons with diabetes [21]. PERL power calculations were based on a projected GFR rate of loss of 3 mL/min/1.73 m^2 in the placebo group and a 2 mL/min/1.73 m^2 rate in the allopurinol-treated group. Given the mean iGFR at baseline of ~68 mL/min/1.73 m^2, this projected benefit would translate into an average delay of progression to ESRD of approximately 8 years. This would be a substantially larger ESRD delay benefit than documented in RASB studies in DN where studies were initiated in subjects with type 1 [3] or type 2 [22, 23] diabetes with, on average, substantially lower baseline GFR.

PERL, which is expected to end in July 2019, will likely represent the first large-scale, placebo-controlled trial of SUA reduction in DN. If successful, PERL will provide proof that higher SUA represents a pathogenetic factor, progression promotor, or both, for DN. If so, early intervention with this safe and inexpensive treatment method could substantially alter the natural history of this single most important renal disease.

Acknowledgements

We thank the National Institutes of Health (NIH/NIDDK UC4DK101108) and the Juvenile Diabetes Research Foundation (JDRF) for their funding of the PERL Study and the entire PERL team for the successful launching of this study.

References

1 USRDS 2016 Annual Data Report. https://www.usrds.org/adr.htm.
2 The DCCT/EDIC Research Group: Intensive diabetes therapy and glomerular filtration rate in type 1 diabetes. N Engl J Med 2011; 365:2366–2376.
3 Lewis EJ, Hunsicker LG, Bain RP, Rohde RD: The effect of angiotensin-converting-enzyme inhibition on diabetic nephropathy. The Collaborative Study Group. N Engl J Med 993; 329:1456–1462.
4 Ali MK, Bullard KM, Saaddine JB, Cowie CC, Imperatore G, Gregg EW: Achievement of goals in U.S. diabetes care, 1999–2010. N Engl J Med 2013;368:1613–1624.
5 Hovind P, Rossing P, Tarnow L, Johnson RJ, Parving HH: Serum uric acid as a predictor for development of diabetic nephropathy in type 1 diabetes: an inception cohort study. Diabetes 2009;58:1668–1671.
6 Pacilli A, Viazzi F, Fioretto P, Giorda C, Ceriello A, Genovese S, Russo G, Guida P, Pontremoli R, De Cosmo S; AMD-Annals Study Group: Epidemiology of diabetic kidney disease in adult patients with T1D in Italy. Diabetes Metab Res Rev 2016, in press.
7 Zoppini G, Targher G, Chonchol M, Ortalda V, Abaterusso C, Pichiri I, Negri C, Bonora E: Serum uric acid levels and incident chronic kidney disease in patients with Type 2 diabetes and preserved kidney function. Diabetes Care 2012;35:99–104.
8 Jalal DI, Rivard CJ, Johnson RJ, Maahs DM, McFann K, Rewers M, Snell-Bergeon JK: Serum uric acid levels predict the development of albuminuria over 6 years in patients with type 1 diabetes. Nephrol Dial Transplant 2010;25:1865–1869.

9 Ahola AJ, Sandholm N, Forsblom C, Harjutsalo V, Dahlström E, Groop PH; FinnDiane Study Group The serum uric acid concentration is not causally linked to diabetic nephropathy in type 1 diabetes. Kidney Int 2017;9:1178–1185.
10 Ficociello LH, Rosolowsky ET, Niewczas MA, Maselli NJ, Weinberg JM, Aschengrau A, Eckfeldt JH, Stanton RC, Galecki AT, Doria A, Warram JH, Krolewski AS: High-normal serum uric acid increases risk of early progressive renal function loss in type 1 diabetes: results of a 6-year follow-up. Diabetes Care 2010;33:1337–1343.
11 Hayashino Y, Okamura S, Tsujii S, Ishii H: Association of serum uric acid levels with the risk of development or progression of albuminuria among Japanese patients with type 2 diabetes. Acta Diabetol 2016;53:599–607.
12 Lytvyn Y, Škrtić M, Yang GK, Yip PM, Perkins BA, Cherney DZ: Glycosuria-mediated urinary uric acid excretion in patients with uncomplicated type 1 diabetes. Am J physiol Renal Physiol 2015;308:F77–F83.
13 Chang YH, Lei CC, Lin KC, Chang DM, Hsieh CH, Lee YJ: Serum uric acid level as an indicator for CKD regression and progression in patients with type 2 diabetes: a 4.6-year cohort study. Diabetes Metab Res Rev 2016;32:557–564.
14 Goicoechea M, de Vinuesa SG, Verdalles U, Ruiz-Caro C, Ampuero J, Rincón A, Arroyo D, Luño J: Effect of allopurinol in chronic kidney disease progression and cardiovascular risk. Clin J Am Soc Nephrol 2010;5:1388–1393.
15 Siu YP, Leung KT, Tong MK, Kwan TH: Use of allopurinol in slowing the progression of renal disease through its ability to lower SUA level. Am J Kidney Dis 2006;47:51–59.
16 Liu P, Chen Y, Wang B, Zhang F, Wang D, Wang Y: Allopurinol treatment improves renal function in patients with type 2 diabetes and asymptomatic hyperuricemia: 3-year randomized parallel-controlled study. Clin Endocrin (Oxf) 2015;83:475–482.
17 Miao Y, Ottenbros SA, Laverman GD, Brenner BM, Cooper ME, Parving HH, Grobbee DE, Shahinfar S, de Zeeuw D, Lambers Heerspink HJ: Effect of a reduction in uric acid on renal outcomes during losartan treatment: a post hoc analysis of the reduction of endpoints in non-insulin-dependent diabetes mellitus with the angiotensin II antagonist losartan trial. Hypertension 2011;58: 2–7.
18 Zinman B, Wanner C, Lachin JM, Fitchett D, Bluhmki E, Hantel S, Mattheus M, Devins T, Johansen OE, Woerle HJ, Broedl UC, Inzucchi SE; EMPA-REG Outcome Investigators: Empagliflozin, cardiovascular outcomes, and mortality in type 2 diabetes. N Engl J Med 2016;373:2117–2128.
19 Wanner C, Inzucchi SE, Lachin JM, Fitchett D, von Eynatten M, Mattheus M, Johansen OE, Woerle HJ, Broedl UC, Zinman B; EMPA-REG Outcome Investigators: Empagliflozin and progression of kidney disease in type 2 diabetes. N Engl J Med 2016;375:323–334.
20 Maahs DM, Caramori L, Cherney DZ, Galecki AT, Gao C, Jalal D, Perkins BA, Pop-Busui R, Rossing P, Mauer M, Doria A; PERL Consortium: Uric acid lowering to prevent kidney function loss in diabetes: the preventing early renal function loss (PERL) allopurinol study. Curr Diab Rep 2013;13:550–559.
21 National Kidney Foundation: KDOQI Clinical Practice Guideline for Diabetes and CKD: 2012 Update. Am J Kidney Dis 2012;60:850–886.
22 Lewis EJ, Hunsicker LG, Clarke WR, Berl T, Pohl MA, Lewis JB, Ritz E, Atkins RC, Rohde R, Raz I; Collaborative Study Group: Renoprotective effect of the angiotensin-receptor antagonist irbesartan in patients with nephropathy due to type 2 diabetes. N Engl J Med 2001;345:851–860.
23 Brenner BM, Cooper ME, de Zeeuw D, Keane WF, Mitch WE, Parving HH, Remuzzi G, Snapinn SM, Zhang Z, Shahinfar S; RENAAL Study Investigators: Effects of losartan on renal and cardiovascular outcomes in patients with type 2 diabetes and nephropathy. N Engl J Med 2001;345:861–869.

Michael Mauer
Department of Pediatrics
2450 Riverside Avenue, East Building, MB68
Minneapolis, MN, 55410 (USA)
E-Mail Mauer002@umn.edu

Treviño-Becerra A, Iseki K (eds): Uric Acid in Chronic Kidney Disease.
Contrib Nephrol. Basel, Karger, 2018, vol 192, pp 110–115 (DOI: 10.1159/000484285)

Uric Acid in Pregnancy: New Concepts

Armando Alberto Moreno Santillan[a] · Jesus Carlos Briones Garduño[b] · Manuel Antonio Diaz de Leon Ponce[c]

[a]Department of Obstetrics, Obstetrics and Gynecology Hospital "Dr. Luis Castelazo Ayala" IMSS, Mexico City, Fellow of the American Congress of Obstetricians and Gynecologist; [b]Member of the National Academy of Medicine, and Mexican Academy of Surgery, Fellow of the American College of Physicians, Mexico City, CMD in Obstetrics and Gynecology Department, General Hospital of Mexico "Dr. Eduardo Liceaga" SSA, Mexico City, [c]Member of the National Academy of Medicine, and Mexican Academy of Surgery, Fellow of the American College of Physicians, Mexico City, Mexico

Abstract

The relationship between hyperuricemia and hypertensive disorders is well established; however, until today, the role of uric acid in the clinical course of severe preeclampsia has not been elucidated. Some recent studies suggest that at the time of presentation, subjects with severe preeclampsia frequently have significantly elevated serum uric acid levels, and that the degree of elevation correlates with the severity of the maternal syndrome and fetal morbimortality. In this chapter, we present our workgroup experience. In 2016, we designed a prospective, cross-sectional comparative study. A sample of 200 patients – 100 with severe preeclampsia and 100 with normotensive pregnancy – was obtained. Plasmatic uric acid levels were recorded in units of mg/dL as clinical variables and as laboratory and fetal growth data. We considered uric acid equal to or more than 6.0 mg/dL as the elevated level. To relate the significance of elevated uric acid levels with variables, chi-square tests and Mann-Whitney U test were applied. Any p value equal or <0.05 was accepted as significant. We found significant difference ($p = 0.05$) between serum uric acid levels among both groups. In comparison with the healthy patients, patients with severe preeclampsia and uric acid greater than 6 mg/dl presented significant differences in relation to fetal complications and maternal laboratory and clinical variables. Our conclusion is that values equal to or greater than 6 mg/dL of serum uric acid in patients with severe preeclampsia may be a valuable biomarker for preeclampsia and an association with the presence of adverse fetal and maternal effects.

Introduction

Uric acid is the final product of purine catabolism by the enzymatic action of the xantine oxidorreductase. This enzyme has two forms that are convertible between them – the xantine oxidase (XO) and the xantine dehydrogenase (XDH). The XO reduces molecular oxygen, while the XDH reduces both oxygen and the NAD+ taking a great affinity for the second substrate. In addition, the XDH is more abundant in vivo and can be converted to XO in an irreversible manner by a variety of enzymes such as trypsin, chymotrypsin, and pancreatin. The liver and the small intestine are the major sources of XO, but currently there is evidence that both the heart and the vascular endothelium express XO. The main enzyme action of the XO is the catalytic conversion of consecutive hypoxanthine to xanthine and then from xanthine to uric acid. As byproducts of these reactions, powerful EROs, molecules that possess high reactivity with other substrates, such as hydrogen peroxide (H_2O_2), and superoxide anion (O2) are formed. Uric acid is mainly secreted by the kidneys and its plasma concentration depends on the pH of the urine, urine volume, body volume, renal function, diet, and use of certain medications [1–3].

During normal pregnancy, maternal physiological adaptations occur and many biochemical measurements deviate from the normal range for non-pregnant females. In normal pregnancy, maternal uric acid levels decrease by 25–35% during the first trimester; this phenomenon can be explained by the expansion in blood volume, increased renal blood flow, increased glomerular filtration rate, and the uricosuric action of estrogen. During the later weeks of pregnancy, uric acid is reabsorbed in increasing amounts and the maternal serum concentrations increase again. The placenta, in normal pregnancy, is a source of purines, which also explains the reason for the physiologic increase in the levels of uric acid [4, 5].

Pregnancies complicated by hypertension are sometimes associated with marked increases in maternal serum uric acid levels. The association between hyperuricemia with preeclampsia is known since 1917 and the relationship between the degree of hyperuricemia and the severity of the preeclampsia was described in 1934. Since then there have been several studies on the role of uric acid in the progression of preeclampsia; however, until our days, the participation of uric acid in the pathophysiology and clinical evolution of preeclampsia has been controversial. The relationship between uric acid and the development of arterial hypertension not related to pregnancy is perfectly established, so that in addition to being considered a biomarker of hypertension, it is also believed that it has an important role to play in its etiology [6–8].

It is believed that uric acid increases with the progression of preeclampsia due to a combination of several factors such as the decrease of the glomerular filtration, the endothelial lesion, and the proinflammatory state. There is evidence that demonstrates the relationship between uric acid and the endothelial dysfunction, which is characteristic of the preeclampsia [2, 3].

Some of the actions of the uric acid that contribute to the endothelial dysfunction during the preeclampsia are as follows:

- Potent inhibitor of the endothelial function [3].
- Locks the role of VEGF [9].
- Inhibits the trophoblastic invasion in vitro [3, 9].
- Stimulates the inflammatory response by stimulating the interleukin-1, interleukin-6 and tumor necrosis factor-alpha [2].

The presence of high levels of uric acid in the first trimester has been associated with 3.22 times increased risk of gestational hypertension and preeclampsia. Based on the above details, it has been postulated that the presence of uric acid in the preeclamptic patient is not only a biomarker but also a contributor to the pathogenesis of preeclampsia [2, 5–8].

Several studies have linked high levels of uric acid to the increased risk of fetal morbidity and mortality. In women with pregnancy hypertensive disease, uric acid levels correlate with the pulsatility index of the umbilical artery and the middle cerebral artery. There is also a correlation between levels of uric acid and acid parameters fetal bases. The fetuses exposed to hypoxia (a decrease of the placental perfusion) have elevated serum levels of metabolites of the purine [8–11].

The relationship between hyperuricemia and hypertensive disorders has been well established; however, until our days, the involvement of uric acid in the pathophysiology and clinical evolution of severe preeclampsia has not been clarified. The measurement of uric acid is a test within the reach of most of the hospital centers, so that to define its role in severe preeclampsia can have a high impact on the patients with this pathology [11–13].

Description of Our Experience

Our workgroup designed a prospective, cross-sectional, and comparative study. In the present study, we randomly included 200 patients who were treated in the department of obstetrics in the Hospital "Dr. Luis Castelazo Ayala" IMSS and in the General Hospital of Mexico "Dr. Eduardo Liceaga" SSA, Mexico. Of the total number of patients, 100 had a diagnosis of severe preeclampsia and 100 were healthy patients with normal pregnancy. We excluded patients with pregnancy of less than 20 weeks of gestation or with concomitant diseases. Approximately 5 mL of peripheral blood were extracted from each patient for measuring uric

Table 1. Laboratory values between groups

Parameter	Healthy pregnancy (n = 100)	Severe preeclampsia (n = 100)	p value*
Uric acid	3.99±0.77	5.43±1.38	0.05
Creatinine	0.64±0.5	0.72±0.22	0.05
GOT	18.6±34	25.9±129	0.05
GPT	31.5±60.7	40.1±108	0.05
LD	52.8±55	205.52±136.4	0.05
DB	0.09±0.14	0.07±0.143	0.01
IB	0.22±0.14	0.22±0.2	ns
TB	0.32±0.18	0.32±0.3	ns
Platelets	194.646±73.530	155.700±125.810	0.05
Hemoglobin	12.2±1.7	11.97±4.32	0.05
Leukocytes	8.8±2.92	9.2±22.3	ns

GOT, glutamic oxaloacetic transaminase; GPT, glutamic pyruvic transaminase; LD, Lactate dehydrogenase; DB, direct bilirubin; IB, indirect bilirubin; TB, total bilirubin; ns, not significant. * Mann-Whitney U.

acid. The presence of more than 6.0 mg/dL of uric acid was considered increased levels. We defined adverse fetal results as the presence of one or more of the following nominal variables:

- Apgar score less than or equal to 6 at birth or at 5 min.
- Acute fetal complications.
- Respiratory distress syndrome.

From each group, we described the general characteristics and the measures of central tendency (average, fashion, and median) and measures of dispersion (range and standard deviation) for their statistical analysis. To relate the significance of uric acid levels with the dependent variables, we applied the tests of χ^2 and Mann-Whitney U. $p < 0.05$ was accepted as significant. The statistical analysis was realized with the STATA program version 12.0 (StataCorp, College Station, TX, USA).

We found significant differences between the values of uric acid ($p = 0.05$), creatinine, glutamic oxaloacetic transaminase, glutamic pyruvic transaminase, lactate dehydrogenase, direct bilirubin, platelets, and hemoglobin, between the 2 groups (Table 1).

Details regarding the distribution between patients with diagnosis of severe preeclampsia with increased uric acid and healthy patients, as well as its relationship with fetal, maternal, and clinical and laboratory variables are presented in Table 2.

Table 2. Healthy and severe preeclampsia patients with uric acid >6 mg/dL

Variable	Healthy pregnancy with UA >6 mg/dL, *n*	Severe preeclampsia with UA >6 mg/dL, *n*	*p* value*
Fetal variables			
Apgar at 1 min <6	1	12	0.05
Prematurity (<34 weeks)	4	17	0.05
Admission to intensive care unit	2	16	0.05
Death	0	1	ns
Intrauterine growth restriction	0	4	0.001
Respiratory distress syndrome	4	18	0.05
Maternal clinical variables			
SBP >160 mm Hg	1	18	0.05
DBP >90 mm Hg	4	23	0.05
Maternal bleeding >500 mL	11	17	ns
Laboratory values			
Platelets <100,000/mm^3	2	10	0.05
GOT >70 IU/L	2	7	0.001
GPT >70 IU/L	4	13	0.05
LD >600 IU/L	0	3	0.006
Creatinine >1.2 mg/dL	1	2	ns
Urine proteins >300 mg/dL	0	8	0.05

* Chi-square.
UA, uric acid; SBP, systolic blood pressure; DBP, diastolic blood pressure; GOT, glutamic oxaloacetic transaminase; GPT, glutamic pyruvic transaminase; LD, lactate dehydrogenase; ns, not significant.

Analysis of the data revealed that there is a significant difference between the levels of uric acid in patients with severe preeclampsia when compared to those in the group of healthy patients.

One of the more interesting findings was that in comparison with the healthy patients, patients with severe preeclampsia and with uric acid levels greater than 6 mg/dL presented significant differences in relation to fetal complications as prematurity, Apgar score less than 6 points at one minute of birth, entrance to neonatal intensive care unit, presence of respiratory distress syndrome, or intrauterine growth restriction; we also found significant difference in maternal complications such as the presence of systolic blood pressure higher than 160 mm Hg and blood pressure higher than 90 mm Hg; as well as the alteration of laboratory values such as platelet count lower than 100,000/mm^3, GTO >70 IU/L, glutamic pyruvic transaminase IU/L >70, lactate dehydrogenase >600 UI/L, and urine proteins >300 mg/dL.

Conclusion

For more than a 100 years, the clinical utility of the uric acid has been widely discussed and several national and international studies have shown conflicting results, so that their role had been relegated in recent years; however, the present study and the growing current evidence on the role of uric acid in the pathophysiology of preeclampsia forces us to reevaluate its the role, not only as a prognostic marker but also as a part of the complex pathogenesis of preeclampsia itself.

On the basis of our results, we can state that the measurement of uric acid is a test that should be requested as a routine protocol study of the patients with severe preeclampsia. The finding of a value of uric acid greater than 6 mg/dL in the patient with severe preeclampsia should alert on the possibility of maternal and fetal complications, so the obstetrician must consider the use of allopurinol to reduce the serum and urinary uric acid concentrations and all the potential complications.

References

1 Alcaino H, Greig D, Castro P, et al: Uric acid: a molecule with a paradoxical actions in heart failure. Rev Med Chile 2011;139:505–515.

2 Bainbridge SA, Roberts JM: Uric acid as a pathogenic factor in preeclampsia. Placenta 2008;29(suppl A):S67–S72.

3 Anceschi MM, Piazze JJ, Maranghi L, et al: Maternal serum uric acid as predictor of fetal acidemia. Int Jour Gyn Obst 2002;77:35–36.

4 Martin AC, Brown MA: Could uric acid have a pathogenic role in pre-eclampsia? Nat Rev Nephrol 2010;6:744–748.

5 Lam C, Lim KH, Kang DH, Karumanchi SA: Uric acid and preeclampsia. Semin Nephrol 2005;25:56–60.

6 Powers WR, Bodnar LM, Ness RB, et al: Uric acid concentrations in early pregnancy among preeclamptic women with gestational hyperuricemia at delivery. Am J Obstet Gynecol 2006;194:160.e1–e8.

7 Chappell LC, Seed PT, Briley A, Kelly FJ, Hunt BJ, Charnock-Jones DS, et al: A longitudinal study of biochemical variables in women at risk of preeclampsia. Am J Obstet Gynecol 2002;187:127–136.

8 Laughon SK, Catov J, Powers RW: First trimester uric acid and adverse pregnancy outcomes. Am J Hypertens 2011;24:489–495.

9 Johnson RJ, Kanbay M, Kang DH: Uric acid: a clinically useful marker to distinguish preeclampsia from gestational hypertension. Hypertension 2011;58:548–549.

10 Schackis RC: Hyperuricaemia and preeclampsia: is there a pathogenic link? Med Hypotheses 2004;63:239–244.

11 Vazquez-Rodriguez JG, Rico-Trejo EI: [Role of uric acid in preeclampsia-eclampsia]. Obstet Ginecol Mex 2011;79:292–297.

12 Moreno SAA, Paz CD, Briones GJC, Díaz de León PM: Relation of hyperuricemia with maternal and perinatal complications in severe preeclampsia. EC Gynaecology 2016;3:235–242.

13 Brien ME, Duval C, Palacios J, et al: Uric acid crystals induce placental inflammation and alter trophoblast function via an IL-1-dependent pathway: implications for fetal growth restriction. J Immunol 2017;198:443–451.

Manuel Antonio Diaz de León Ponce
Naranjo 94-303
Colonia Santa Maria al Ribera, Delegacion Cuauhtemoc
Mexico City (Mexico)
E-Mail manueldeleonponce@hotmail.com

Treviño-Becerra A, Iseki K (eds): Uric Acid in Chronic Kidney Disease.
Contrib Nephrol. Basel, Karger, 2018, vol 192, pp 116–124 (DOI: 10.1159/000484286)

Uric Acid Renal Lithiasis: New Concepts

Fabiola Pazos Pérez

Department of Nephrology, Specialty Hospital, National Medical Center XXI Century, Mexico City, Mexico

Abstract

Background: Uric acid (UA) stones are responsible for 5–10% of the formation of all kidney stones. Recently, an association between UA stones and insulin resistance, diabetes mellitus, and obesity has been demonstrated and so the incidence has increased. The development of UA stones is dependent on several risk factors, including genetic predisposition, geographical location, dietary indiscretion, and various metabolic characteristics. ***Summary:*** UA nephrolithiasis can arise from diverse etiologies, all with distinct underlying defects converging to one or more of 3 defects of hyperuricosuria, acidic urine pH, and low urinary volume. Low urinary pH is the commonest and by far the most important factor in UA nephrolithiasis, but the reason for this defect is unknown. Patients with UA nephrolithiasis have normal acid-base parameters assessed according to conventional clinical tests. Studies have revealed that there could be an insufficient production of urinary ammonium buffer. Many transport proteins are candidate participants in urate handling, with URAT1 and GLUT9 being the best characterized to date. Because low urine pH is the most important pathogenic factor of UA stone formation, urine alkalinization is an effective intervention to reduce UA crystallization and dissolve UA stones. ***Key Messages:*** Epidemiological and metabolic studies have indicated an association between UA nephrolithiasis and insulin resistance. Some potential mechanisms include impaired ammoniagenesis caused by resistance to insulin action in the renal proximal tubule or due to substrate competition by free fatty acids. The identification of novel complementary DNA has provided an interesting insight into the renal handling of UA, including one genetic cause of renal UA wasting.

Epidemiology

Although many articles indicate that uric acid (UA) stones represent about 5–10% of all kidney stones formation, they are the third most common urinary stones after calcium oxalate and struvite stones. There are wide regional differences in the incidence of UA containing stones. For example, prevalence is highest in the Middle East (22–28%) and in the United States, it is only 8–10% [1]. The exact cause for global diversity in UA lithiasis prevalence has not yet been fully elucidated. This maybe because there is a tendency in the literature to collectively include all UA containing stone formers into a single category [2]; another reason could be a high prevalence of obesity or metabolic syndrome, diabetes, and hypertension that are commonly associated with UA nephrolithiasis. It has been established that stones formers with metabolic syndrome or with type 2 diabetes have UA with a higher prevalence than other populations [3]. Pak et al. [4] reported that 33.9% of 59 stone-forming patients with type 2 diabetes had UA stones as compared with only 6.2% among non-diabetic stone formers.

Pathophysiology of UA Stone Formation

Physical Chemistry of UA

Humans excrete urea primarily although there is some UA excretion due to the unusual lack of uricase. Ammonia has the dual role of carrying nitrogen and acting as H+ acceptor in urine and thus sets the urinary pH. The UA and ammonia system can be poised to cause UA precipitation. UA is an end product of purine metabolism. It is formed from the degradation of nucleic acid via hypoxanthine and xanthine in the presence of xanthine oxidase. In other mammals, UA is further converted into allantoin by enzyme uricase. UA has limited solubility, while allantoin is highly soluble in water; that is why man is prone to UA stone formation, while other mammals do not form these stones [5]. The pKa of UA is 5.75 in urine at 37°C. Thus, 50% of UA is in an undissociated or insoluble form and 50% in dissociated or soluble form at this pH (monosodium urate). Urinary pH determines the balance between UA and urate; as urinary pH reaches 6.5, most of the UA is in the more soluble monosodium urate form [6]. Urinary pH determines the balance between UA and urate. The solubility of monosodium urate is determined by the urinary cationic environment. Studies have shown that potassium increases the solubility of urate and sodium decreases it [7]. The consequent fall in UA dissociation reduces UA solubility, leading to the urinary supersaturation and crystallization of UA. At a pH of 5.35, 200 mg/L of UA is soluble before becoming supersaturated, whereas at a pH of 6.5 over 1,200 mg/L can be present and not exceed solubility. After UA crystals precipitate, the subsequent mechanism(s) for UA stone formation remain unclear. The role of urinary inhibitors such as glycosaminoglycans and crystal adhesion to the surface of kidney epithelial cells needs further investigation [8].

Renal Handling of UA

The classic model of UA transport in the human kidney was developed in the 1970s. This involved 4 distinct components: glomerular filtration of virtually all circulating urate, reabsorption of 98–100% of the filtered urate, secretion of up to half of this amount, and postsecretory reabsorption [9]. We now know that in human kidney, renal urate handling involves a complex interplay of urate glomerular filtration followed by a complex array of reabsorptive and secretory mechanisms taking place in the proximal tubule. In the last years, different types of potential urate transporters have been cloned. The urate/anion exchanger URAT1 (*SLC22A12* gene), reabsorbs urate at the apical membrane and is responsible for voltage-driven urate efflux from the proximal tubule. Strong evidence suggests that URAT1 is the major luminal pathway for urate reabsorption in humans. Available evidence suggests that Glucose transporter family member SLC2A9 (GLUT9) may be the principal pathway of basolateral urate exit from the proximal tubule cell in the human kidney [10]. Three multi-specific organic anion transporters – OAT1 and OAT3 localized in the apical membrane of epithelial cells from the proximal tubule and OAT4 (basolateral side) – there is lower affinity than URAT1, although level and type of evidence for a role in renal urate transport is still moderate. Other transporters have been identified, but their role in renal UA management is still controversial [11].

Pathophysiology of Lithogenesis by UA

Intrinsic Factors Associated

Several risk factors have been implicated in the pathogenesis of UA nephrolithiasis, but the underlying mechanisms are not completely understood.

Age and Sex: According to several studies, UA calculi increased with age in both sexes after the age of 50 ; some included predominance in men [12].

Diet: The increase in animal proteins has been associated with an increase in the incidence of urinary acid lithiasis. Diet is low in fiber because fiber decreases the adsorption of sucrose and proteins of animal origin. Low-carbohydrate high-protein diets used for weight reduction, deliver an exaggerated acid load to the kidney, thereby reducing urinary pH and increasing the propensity for UA stone formation [13].

Extrinsic Factors Associated

Low Urinary pH

From the physicochemical viewpoint, one can appreciate that urinary pH is the most important factor for UA precipitation. Most patients with idiopathic UA stones have normal UA excretion, but almost all have a persistently low urine pH that promotes UA precipitation [14]. The pathogenetic mechanism for excessive urine acidity in UA stone-formers is heterogeneous and is in large part unknown. In a small series of patients, ammonium was found to be diminished with increased urine hydrogen ion concentration. Sakhaee et al. [15] studied steady-state urinary acidification parameters while on controlled metabolic diets and demonstrated lower 24-h urinary pH and a lower fraction of urinary net acid excretion as ammonium in UA stone-formers, when compared with normal volunteers and calcium oxalate stone-formers. In addition, UA nephrolithiasis patients displayed a more blunted increase in ammonium ion/ammonia excretion when compared with controls during acute oral acid loading. There is evidence that supports the fact that a circadian cycle variation in urine pH relates to gastric acid secretion; luminal acid extrusion results in base exit from the parietal cells, resulting in a transient alkalinization of the blood, and secondarily of the urine. Although non-stone formers also develop acid urine intermittently, the periodic alkalinization of urine appears to be sufficient to protect them from forming UA stones [16].

Another process that could lead to an excessively high level of UA in UA nephrolithiasis is decreased urinary ammonium. Theories suggest that the conversion of glutamine to alpha-ketoglutarate is impaired, resulting in decreased ammonia production, and in increased purine biosynthesis and degradation, with resulting hyperuricemia. At this time, there are insufficient data to attribute defective ammoniagenesis to decreased glutamine metabolism [17].

Low Urine Volume

The physicochemestry of supersaturation is of great importance, since the concentration rather than the amount of crystallizing solutes is what ultimately establishes stone formation. Reduced urinary volume will amplify the saturation of all solutes and raise the risk of stone formation. Additionally, low volume promotes urinary stasis. Low urine volume can result from inadequate intake or excessive loss of liquid through intestinal tract or excessive sweating [18].

Hyperuricosuria

Hyperuricosuria can be from hyperproduction, dietary intake, or mutations in any renal urate transporters. A given disease can cause UA precipitation via a combination of the low urine volume and low urinary pH.

Etiology
The etiologies for UA stone formation are diverse and complex. Stones can develop as a result of congenital or acquired causes, or can be idiopathic. Congenital disorders may affect UA metabolism or renal tubular urate transport. Acquired causes frequently influence urinary volume, pH, or UA concentration. A UA versus a UA-containing calcium oxalate stone might show quite different underlying pathophysiology, such as the presence of hypercalciuria [19].

Genetic Risk
Ombra et al. [20] identified a possible genetic basis for this increased risk by studying a homogeneous population with a high incidence of UA stones in Sardinia. The *ZNF365* gene on chromosome 10q21–q22 was discovered to be associated with UA nephrolithiasis. Nevertheless, replication studies are required to investigate the involvement of these regions in the genetic contribution to UA stone formation.

Several renal diseases are associated with hyperuricosuria and UA nephrolithiasis, including Fanconi syndrome, Hartnup disease, Wilson's disease, and familial hypouricemic hyperuricosuria. These conditions predispose patients to renal wasting of UA. The identification of the UA transporter URAT1 was a breakthrough in our understanding of urate handling by the nephron, and it is the transporter that is defective in familial hypouricemic hyperuricosuria. To date, 11 different loss-of function mutations have been identified [21].

Most patients with primary gout hyperuricemia have an absolute or relative impairment of renal urate excretion, whereas only a minority present with increased production. UA stone disease can occur at any time in the course of gout in ranges from 10 to 20%. In the primary gout, there is a defect in renal acidification. It is believed that a defect in renal ammoniogenesis is responsible for the decrease in urinary pH, since some studies have evidenced urinary levels of normal urinary nitrate, sulfate, and potassium in these patients. Another characteristic is the increase of tubular adsorption of UA that contributes to the development of hyperuricemia However, calcium oxalate stones are the most common types of stones formed in individuals with gout similar to the way they are formed in individuals without gout [22].

Inborn errors of metabolism, such as hypoxanthine guanine phosphoribosyl transferase deficiency and type 1 collagen storage disease, can cause UA stones because they cause hyperuricemia and hyperuricosuria. HGPRT deficiency results in a failure to salvage purines from cell breakdown, leading to severe hyperuricemia. This condition is X-linked recessive and in its most severe form, Lesch-Nyhan syndrome, is characterized by mental retardation, gout, UA nephrolithiasis, and self-mutilation. Type 1 collagen storage disease, also known as von Gierke disease, is an autosomal recessive defect in glucose-6-phosphatase and affected patients have hypoglycemia, hyperlactacidemia, and hyperuricemia [23].

Gouty Diathesis
An idiopathic form of nephrolithiasis has been described, which develops in the absence of secondary causes. Lithiais are presented in pure form or associated with calcium oxalate with low urinary pH (less than 5.5). This form is described as "gout diathesis." Hyperuricemia is not considered a characteristic for the diagnosis of gout diathesis, because in the latent phase, some patients have normouricemia. This entity has not been well accepted due to the fact that this specific physiopathology is not elucidated. The diagnostic criterion of pH is still not enough because there are patients who despite maintaining urinary pH below 5.5 do not develop lithiasis and patients with lithiasis who do not have low pH [24].

Secondary Causes
Metabolic Syndrome, Diabetes Mellitus, and Insulin Resistance. Studies have emphasized the increasing importance of insulin resistance in the pathogenesis of UA stones. Diabetics have 20–30% of UA stones than those in the general population. Physiologic experiments have shown that acute surges in insulin elevate urinary pH by stimulating proximal renal tubular ammoniagenesis by increasing catabolism of glutamine into 2 molecules of ammonia and α-ketoglutarate as well as the activity of the sodium/hydrogen ion exchanger 3 that secretes and traps ammonia in the urinary space as ammonium [25]. In some animal models, elevated levels of free fatty acids (often observed in insulin-resistant states) increase levels of acetyl-CoA, which competes with α-ketoglutarate for entry into the Krebs cycle. Decreased metabolism α-ketoglutarate leads to its accumulation and in turn impedes the catabolism of glutamine by the mass-law effect, effectively reducing ammoniagenesis [26].

Neoplastic Disorders. Those with myeloproliferative disorders and malignancy may have elevated levels of UA in the blood from rapid cell turnover and tumor necrosis, especially in the setting of chemotherapy. Along with the electrolyte abnormalities that occur during tumor lysis, massive hyperuricemia and hyperuricosuria may occur, leading to urate nephropathy. Other conditions associated with a higher incidence of UA nephrolithiasis include conditions with high cell turnover, such as sickle cell disease, hemolytic anemias, polycythemia vera, and psoriasis [27].

Gastrointestinal Disorders: Gastrointestinal losses of alkali are commonly associated with systemic metabolic acidosis, a low urine pH, hypocitraturia, and low urine volumes, which predispose to both UA and calcium oxalate stones.

Examples include intestinal fistulas, or certain types of chronic (inflammatory bowel disease) or osmotic diarrhea due to water-soluble solutes such as magnesium, lactulose, and polyethylene glycol [26, 27].

Uricosuric Drugs: A large number of drugs affect the serum concentration of UA. Some drugs decreased UA excretion for a block of transport proteins involved in urate handling in proximal tubule. Within the group are found diuretics (loop and thiazide types), pyrazinamide, b-blockers, lactic acid, cyclosporine, tacrolimus, theophyline, levodopa, rivabirin, ritonavir, filgastrim, rituximab, basiliximab, and sildenafil. Drugs that increased UA production by accelerated purine nucleotide degradation or for increased turnover rate of cell death are salicylates (high doses), losartan, nifedipine, trimetoprim-sulfamethoxazole, amlodipino, fenofibrate, atorvastatin, rosuvastatin, estrogens, vitamin C, dicoumarol, calcitonin, and sevelamer. In addition, some drugs shows "biphasic effect," which causes hyperuricemia in lower doses but hypouricemia in larger doses, like salicylate. However, some hypouricemic agents may induce nephrolithiasis by a significant increase in UA excretion [28].

Management and Treatment

Unlike the other main stone types, UA stones can be managed medically. The aim of the treatment is to increase the solubility of UA in urine and to reduce its concentration.

Increased Fluid Intake

Increasing urine volume to 2.5–3.0 L/day is essential and should be emphasized.

Diet

Protein confers acid and other possible lithogenic factors. The effect is more pronounced in animal than in plant proteins partly as a result of higher acid content per gram of animal protein. Protein restriction raises urinary citrate by acting on the renal proximal tubule. These increased urinary pH and reduced the formation of UA lithos. Fruits with high potassium content provide organic anions that will be metabolized to alkali. Alkali in fruits effectively neutralizes the acid load delivered by animal proteins [29].

Alcalinization with Potassium Citrate

This treatment creates a urinary environment less conducive to the crystallization of UA by increasing urinary pH and reducing the amount of undissociated UA. It inhibits urinary crystallization of calcium oxalate by reducing urinary saturation and augmenting inhibitor activity owing to the rise in urinary citrate and pH. Other forms of alkali, such as sodium citrate or sodium bicarbonate, are less ideal because the sodium load worsens hypercalciuria and increases sodium urate saturation [30].

Efficacy of Xanthine Oxidase Inhibitors
Xanthine oxidase inhibitors are usually reserved for patients who continue to have stones despite urinary alkalinization and a prescribed higher fluid intake.

Conclusions

A thorough understanding of the epidemiology and pathophysiology of UA nephrolithiasis is crucial for the diagnosis, treatment, and prevention of stones in patients. The pathogenesis of UA nephrolithiasis involves hyperuricosuria, low urinary volume, and acid urine pH. These conditions drive the conversion of the relatively soluble urate salt into insoluble UA. Nevertheless, the most important biochemical risk factor is a persistently low urine pH and hyperuricosuria is not always present in patients with pure UA stones. Common clinical conditions that increase the risk of UA stone formation include gout, chronic diarrhea, diabetes, and the metabolic syndrome.

In patients with UA nephrolithiasis, urinary alkalinization with potassium citrate is recommended more than sodium citrate or bicarbonate with an increased fluid intake. Xanthine oxidase inhibitors are usually reserved for patients who continue to have stones despite urinary alkalinization and a prescribed higher fluid intake. Invasive treatments may be needed for large and acutely symptomatic stones.

The recognition of metabolic, molecular, and genetic factors that influence urinary pH, and UA metabolism and excretion will provide novel insights into the pathogenesis of UA stones and open the way for the formulation of new therapeutic strategies.

References

1 Sakhaee K: Epidemiology and clinical pathophysiology of uric acid kidney stones. J Nephrol 2014;27:241–245.
2 Scholz D, Schwille PO, Ulbrich D, et al: Composition of renal stones and their frequency in a stone clinic: relationship to parameters of mineral metabolism in serum and urine. Urol Res 1979;7:161–170.
3 Daudon M, Lacour B, Jungers P: High prevalence of uric acid calculi in diabetic stone formers. Nephrol Dial Transplant 2005;20: 468–469.
4 Pak CYC, Sakhaee K, Moe O, Preminger GM, Poindexter JR, Peterson RD, Pietrow P, Ekeruo W: Biochemical profile of stone-forming patients with diabetes mellitus. Urology 2003;61:523–527.

5 Halperin ML, Jungas RL: Metabolic production and renal disposal of hydrogen ions. Kidney Int 1983;24:709–713.
6 Moe OW, Abate N, Sakhaee K: Pathophysiology of uric acid nephrolithiasis. Endocrinol Metab Clin N Am 2002;31:895–914.
7 Sakhaee K, Nicar M, Hill K, Hill K, Pak CY: Contrasting effects of potassium citrate and sodium citrate therapies on urinary chemistries and crystallization of stone-forming salts. Kidney Int 1983;24:348–352.
8 Koka RM, Huang E, Lieske JC: Adhesion of uric acid crystals to the surface of renal epithelial cells. Am J Physiol 2000;278:F989–F998.
9 Gutman AB, Yu TF, Berger L: Tubular secretion of urate in man. J Clin Invest 1959;38: 1778–1781.
10 Bobulescu IA, Moe OW: Renal transport of uric acid: evolving concepts and uncertainties. Adv Chronic Kidney Dis 2012;19:358–371.
11 So A, Thorens B: Uric acid transport and disease. J Clin Invest 2010;120:1791–1799.
12 Lieske JC, Rule AD, Krambeck AE, Williams JC, Bergstralh EJ, Mehta RA, Moyer TP: Stone composition as a function of age and sex. Clin J Am Soc Nephrol 2014;9:2141–2146.
13 Fry C, Sellaturay S: The metabolic basis for urolithiasis. Surgery 2008;26:136–140.
14 Henneman PH, Wallach S, Dempsey E: The metabolic defect responsible for uric acid stone formation. J Clin Invest 1962;61:537–542.
15 Sakhaee K, Adams-Huet B, Moe OW, Pak CY: Pathophysiologic basis for normouricosuric uric acid nephrolithiasis. Kidney Int 2002;62:971–979.
16 Niv Y, Fraser GM: The alkaline tide phenomenon. J Clin Gastroenterol 2002;35:5–8.
17 Gutman A, Yu T: An abnormality of glutamine metabolism in primary gout. Am J Med 1963;35:820–831.
18 Moe OW: Kidney stones: pathophysiology and medical management. Lancet 2006;367: 333–344.
19 Seegmiller JE, Grayzel AI, Laster L, Liddle L: Uric acid production in gout. J Clin Invest 1961;40:1304–1314.
20 Ombra MN, Forabosco P, Casula S, Angius A, Maestrale G, Petretto E, Casu G, Colussi G, Usai E, Melis P, Pirastu M: Identification of a new candidate locus for uric acid nephrolithiasis. Am J Hum Genet 2001;63:1119–1129.
21 Pak CY, Poindexter JR, Adams-Huet B, Pearle MS: Predictive value of kidney stone composition in the detection of metabolic abnormalities. Am J Med 2003;115:26–32.
22 Rieselbach RE, Sorensen LB, Shelp WD, Steele TH: Disminished urate secretion per nephron as a basis for primary gout. Ann Intern Med 1970;73:359–366.
23 Ngo TC, Assumes DG: Uric acid nephrolithiasis: recent progress and future directions. Rev Urol 2007;9:17–27.
24 Khatchadourian J, Preminger GM, Whitson PA, Adams-Huet B, Pak CY: Clinical and biochemical presentation of gouty diathesis: comparison of uric acid versus pure calcium stone formation. J Urol 1995;154:1665–1669.
25 Abate N, Chandalia M, Cabo-Chan AV Jr, Moe OW, Sakhaee K: The metabolic syndrome and uric acid nephrolithiasis: novel features of renal manifestation of insulin resistance. Kidney Int 2004;65:386–392.
26 Vinay P, Lemieux G, Cartier P, Ahmad M: Effect of fatty acids on renal ammoniagenesis in in vivo and in vitro studies. Am J Physiol 1976;231:880–887.
27 Tsimberidou AM, Keating MJ: Hyperuricemic syndromes in cancer patients. Contrib Nephrol 2005;147:47–60.
28 Moriwaki Y: Effects on uric acid metabolism of the drugs except the antihyperuricemics. J Bioequiv Availab 2014;6:10–17.
29 Taylor EN, Stampfer MJ, Curhan GC: Dietary factors and the risk of incident kidney stones in men: new insights after 14 years of follow-up. J Am Soc Nephrol 2004;15:3225–3232.
30 Pak CY, Sakhaee K, Fuller C: Successful management of uric acid nephrolithiasis with potassium citrate. Kidney Int 1986;30:422–428.

Fabiola Pazos Pérez
Department of Nephrology, Specialty Hospital, National Medical Center XXI Century
Cuahutemoc 330 Avenue, Colony Doctors, Delegation Miguel Hidalgo
06720, Mexico City (Mexico)
E-Mail drapazos.nefro@gmail.com

Treviño-Becerra A, Iseki K (eds): Uric Acid in Chronic Kidney Disease.
Contrib Nephrol. Basel, Karger, 2018, vol 192, pp 125–134 (DOI: 10.1159/000484287)

Clinical Significance of Serum Uric Acid Levels in Mexican Young Adults

Araceli Alegría-Díaz[a] · Rafael Valdez-Ortiz[a] · Miguel Murguía-Romero[b, c] · Rafael Jiménez-Flores [b, c] · Rafael Villalobos-Molina [b, c] · Srinivas Mummidi[d] · Ravindranth Duggirala[d] · Juan C. López-Alvarenga[d, e] · Monserrat Pérez-Navarro[a]

[a]Department of Nephrology, Hospital General de México, México City, [b]Iztacala School of Graduate Studies, National Autonomous University of Mexico (FES-I. UNAM), Tlalnepantla, [c]National Laboratory in Health: Molecular Diagnosis and Environmental Effect in Chronic-Degenerative Diseases, National Autonomous University of Mexico (UNAM), Tlalnepantla, México; [d]South Texas Diabetes and Obesity Institute, University of Texas Rio Grande Valley, Edinburg, TX, USA; [e]Universidad Mexico Americana del Norte, Reynosa Tamaulipas, México

Abstract

Background: High serum uric acid concentration (SUA >6 for women [W] or 7 mg/dL for men [M]) in adults is an independent risk factor for causing cardiovascular disease and chronic kidney disease (CKD); the risk of high SUA in young population is still being debated. ***Summary:*** We conducted an epidemiological study to determine the association between SUA quartiles with cardiometabolic risk factors (CRF) and renal impairment in apparently healthy young adults. CRF (dyslipidemia, overweight [Ow], obesity [Ob], blood pressure [BP], hyperglycemia, insulin resistance [IR]) and renal impairment were defined as glomerular filtration rate (GFR) by CKD-Epidemiology Collaboration formula >130/120, <90 mL/min/1.73 m^2, and proteinuria were measured in 18- to 25-year-old students (total n = 5,531). Adjusted ORs by sex were calculated using logistic regression. ***Results:*** The mean SUA was 4.5 ± 1.04 and 6.2 ± 1.2 mg/dL in W and M respectively. High SUA was found in 13.9% (n = 767); prevalence of Ow/Ob 69% (528 of 767), high BP 9% (67), hyperglycemia 15% (112), IR 47% (214), hypertriglyceridemia 35% (269), high LDL-c 16% (120), low HDL-c 52% (399), and metabolic syndrome 33% (249). Prevalence of high GFR was 13% (103), low GFR 8% (62) and proteinuria 5% (37). All risk factors showed a positive relationship with the SUA quartiles with high LDL-c with lowest risk (OR 1.7) and Ow/Ob with highest risk (OR 4.1), independent of sex. ***Key Messages:*** High SUA concentrations (M ≥6.2/W ≥4.5 mg/dL) are associated with CRF and renal impairment in young adults. It is necessary to reevaluate the cutoff points for UA in young adults.

Introduction

High serum concentration of uric acid (SUA) is an independent risk factor for causing chronic kidney disease (CKD) and is recognized as a cardiometabolic risk factor (CRF) [1–7]. The current recommendation for adult SUA levels is below 6 mg/dL for women (W) and below 7 mg/dL for men (M) [8–9]. Kuwabara et al. [10] found that in a population, 30–85 years old, with SUA between 4.2 and 6.3 mg/dL, and with a slight increase of 1 mg/dL from basal level over a period of 5 years, is associated with impairment of glomerular filtration rate (GFR; OR 3.77, 97% CI 3.35–4.26). Leiba et al. [11] in a recent study found that values between 5.2 and 6.0 mg/dL were positively associated with higher cardiovascular risk or mortality. Most of these studies were conducted in people with existing comorbid conditions such as diabetes, old age, and who were at high risk for cardiovascular disease. However, few studies have evaluated the SUA levels and its association with CRF and altered renal function in apparently healthy young adults [12].

Early adulthood provides a window of opportunity for preventive health care related to lifestyle choices, and universities are a perfect setting for implementing surveillance and preventive measures against development of chronic diseases. There is little evidence worldwide about SUA in young population, including its normal range and its potential association with cardiometabolic or impaired renal function risks. The objective of this study was to determine the strength of association between the concentration of UA and risk CRF and renal disease in Mexican young adults.

Methodology

Study Design and Variables

This cross-sectional epidemiological study included students at the Iztacala School of Graduate Studies, National Autonomous University of Mexico, Mexico City. The study was designed in accordance with the Helsinki Declaration.

Subjects were invited to participate voluntarily for a brief physical examination to record their anthropometric measurements, blood pressure (BP), and blood withdrawal for analysis of glucose, uric acid, lipids, and insulin after 8 h fasting. The following variables were transformed from interval scale to nominal scale: central obesity (Ob) ≥90/80 cm for M/W, overweight or obesity (Ow, according BMI-WHO classification); high BP (SBP, DBP, ≥130/85 mm Hg), hyperglycemia (≥100 mg/dL); hyperuricemia (UA >6/7 mg/dL W/M); hypertriglyceridemia (≥150 mg/dL), low HDL-cholesterol (HDL-c <50/40 mg/dL W/M), high LDL-cholesterol (LDL-c >130 mg/dL), insulin resistance (HOMA-IR, >2.3/2.9 W/M). Metabolic syndrome (MetS) was defined according to the criteria established by the International Diabetes Federation and the American Heart Association/National Heart, Lung, and Blood Institute [13].

GFR was estimated by using the CKD-Epidemiology Collaboration formula; stratifying the values obtained by FGR >130/120 mL/min/1.73 m^2 (M/W), FGR normal ≥90–120/90–130 mL/min/1.73 m^2 (W/M), and FGR <90 mL/min/1.73 m^2. Proteinuria was evaluated with protein-reactive strips (ROCHE, Urisys 2400).The presence of traces or ≥15–500 mg/dL of protein, without the presence of bacteria, nitrites, hemoglobin, or erythrocytes in general urine test was considered positive proteinuria [14].

Statistical Analysis

Subjects were divided and analyzed into quartiles of SUA (Q1: M <5.3 and <3.8 in W; Q2: M 5.3–6.1, W 3.8–4.4; Q3: M 6.2–6.9, W 4.5–5.1; Q4: M ≥7, W ≥5.2 mg/dL). Mean differences between quartiles were estimated with analysis of variance, and post hoc analysis was performed with Gabriel test and a significance level of 0.05. Linear trends of serum uric acid quartiles adjusted by sex were evaluated by Wald test, using logistic regression. Association between the quartiles of UA with cardiometabolic and kidney disease risk factors was evaluated by OR (OR, 95% CI) adjusted by sex using logistic regression. Data were analyzed by SPSS version 22 (IBM Corp., Released 2013. IBM SPSS Statistics for Windows, Version 22.0. Armonk, NY, USA).

Results

Association of Uric Acid According to Sex and Cardiometabolic Factors

Our study included a total of 5,531 apparently healthy young adult subjects (W 68%). The overall mean age was 19 ± 2 and the mean SUA concentrations were 4.5 ± 1.04 mg/dL for W and 6.2 ± 1.2 mg/dL for M. Hyperuricemia was identified in 13.9% (n = 767) of total subjects, (W 8%, M 24%). Among hyperuricemic subjects, the prevalence of Ow/Ob was 69% (n = 528 of 767), SBP/DBP of risk was 9% (n = 67), hyperglycemia was 15% (n = 112), IR was 47% (n = 214), hypertriglyceridemia was 35% (n = 269), high LDL-c was 16% (n = 120), low HDL-c was 52% (n = 399), and MetS was 33% (n = 249). The prevalence of FGR >130/120 mL/min/1.73 m^2 was 13% (n = 103), FGR <90 mL/min/1.73 m^2 8% (n = 62) and proteinuria 5% (n = 37). Table 1 summarizes the clinical, anthropometric, and biochemical variables obtained from all the subjects stratified by sex and uric acid quartiles.

Table 1. Clinical, anthropometric, and biochemical parameters of the population by quartile and sex

	Q1	Q2	Q3	Q4	*p**
Men					
n	373	488	434	486	
Age	19.6±1.8	19.5±1.6	19.5±1.7	19.4±1.6	0.69
WC, cm	79.3±8.5^{d}	81.9±9.8^{c}	84.7±11.06^{b}	90.4±13.1^{a}	<0.001
BMI	22.4±3.3^{d}	23.4±3.6^{c}	24.6±4.0^{b}	26.6±5.03^{a}	<0.001
SBP, mm Hg	112±11^{c}	113±12^{b,c}	115±12^{b}	117±12^{a}	<0.001
DBP, mm Hg	75±8^{c}	76±9^{b,c}	76±9^{b}	79±9^{a}	<0.001
Hemoglobin	16.8±0.9	16.9±0.9	16.9±0.9	17±0.9	0.195
TC, mg/dL	158±27^{c}	160±26^{c}	166±29^{b}	173±36^{a}	<0.001
LDL-c, mg/dL	91±22^{c}	93±22$^{b, c}$	96±24^{b}	101±28^{a}	<0.001
HDL-c, mg/dL	47±9^{c}	46±9$^{b, c}$	45±9^{b}	43±9^{a}	<0.001
Triglycerides, mg/dL	100±44^{c}	108±52^{c}	123±70^{b}	147±140^{a}	<0.001
FPG, mg/dL	90±11^{b}	90±9^{b}	91±9^{b}	93±15^{a}	<0.001
Urea, mg/dL	25.9±7.1^{b}	27.9±6.1$^{a, b}$	28±6.9^{a}	28.5±6.1^{a}	<0.001
Creatinine, mg/dL	0.91±0.1^{c}	0.94±0.11^{b}	0.95±0.11^{b}	0.97±0.15^{a}	<0.001
Insulin, µU/ml	7.4±3.4^{b}	7.4±3.8^{b}	8.6±5^{b}	10.9±6.8^{a}	<0.001
GFR/mL/min/1.73 m^2	119±11^{c}	116±12^{b}	114±13$^{a, b}$	113±14^{a}	<0.001
Women					
n	488	864	896	1,012	
Age	19.2±1.6	19.2±1.6	19±1.5	19±1.5	0.22
WC, cm	76.5±8.2^{d}	78.7±9.57^{c}	81±10.4^{b}	86.1±11.8^{a}	<0.001
BMI	22.3±3.1^{d}	23.08±3.45^{c}	24±4^{b}	26.3±4.8^{a}	<0.001
SBP, mm Hg	103±10^{c}	103±11^{b,c}	105±11^{b}	108±11^{a}	<0.001
DBP, mm Hg	69±9^{c}	70±8^{b,c}	70±8^{b}	73±9^{a}	<0.001
Hemoglobin	14.4±1.1^{c}	14.6±0.9^{b}	14.7±0.9^{b}	14.8±0.9^{a}	<0.001
TC, mg/dL	160±28^{c}	164±29^{b}	166±30^{b}	315±65^{a}	<0.001
LDL-c, mg/dL	90±23^{c}	94±23^{b}	95±25^{b}	101±25^{a}	<0.001
HDL-c, mg/dL	51±10^{c}	50±10$^{b, c}$	49±10^{b}	47±9^{a}	<0.001
Triglycerides, mg/dL	93±37^{d}	100±41^{c}	108±48^{b}	130±63^{a}	<0.001
FPG, mg/dL	87±7^{c}	88±9$^{b, c}$	88±8^{b}	90±8^{a}	<0.001
Urea, mg/dL	21.4±5.7^{c}	22.9±6.2$^{b, c}$	23±5.7^{b}	24.5±6.5^{a}	<0.001
Creatinine, mg/dL	0.74±0.08^{c}	0.75±0.08$^{b, c}$	0.76±0.08^{b}	0.79±0.2^{a}	<0.001
Insulin, µU/mL	8.6±3.3^{c}	9.6±5.1^{c}	10.9±5.8^{b}	13±8.6^{a}	<0.001
GFR/mL/min/1.73 m^2	117±12^{c}	115±12^{b}	114±12^{b}	111±14^{a}	<0.001

Sex-specific quartiles for uric acid (<5.3, 5.3–6.1, 6.2–6.9, ≥7 mg/dL) for men; (<3.8, 3.8-4.4, 4.5–5.1 ≥5.2 mg/dL) for women. Data are means ± SD. SUA, serum uric acid; WC, waist circumference; BMI, body mass index; SBP, systolic blood pressure; DBP, diastolic blood pressure; TC, total cholesterol; LDL-C, low-density lipoprotein cholesterol; HDL-C, high-density lipoprotein cholesterol; FPG, fasting plasma glucose; GFR, glomerular filtration rate. * ANOVA. Post hoc: Gabriel test. The superscript letters show homogeneous groups.

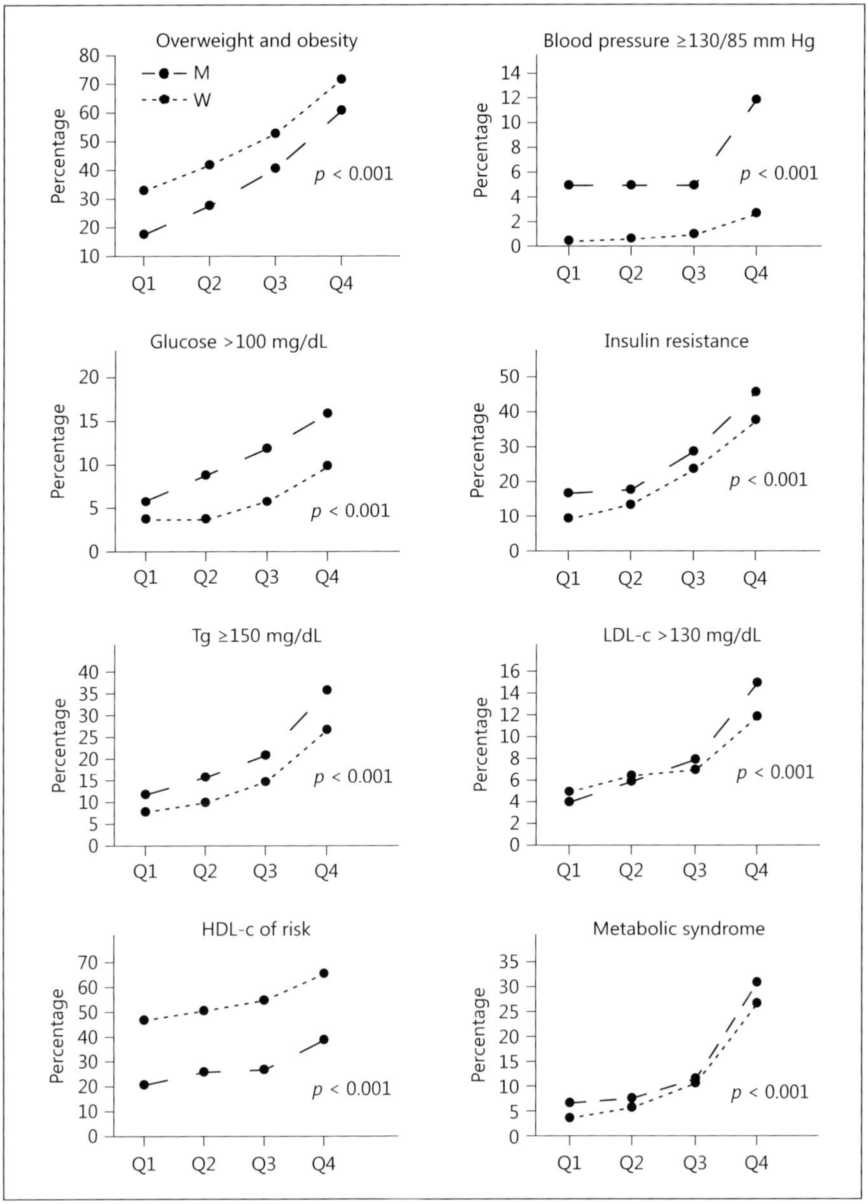

Fig. 1. Relative frequency of cardiometabolic risk factors by quartiles of SUA and sex.

A higher frequency of M showed higher fasting glucose, high BP, hypertriglyceridemia relative to W. In contrast, W had a higher frequency of low HDL-c and GFR >90 mL/min/1.7 m^2 relative to M. There was a positive association with quartiles of SUA and most of the variables as shown in Figure 1 and 2.

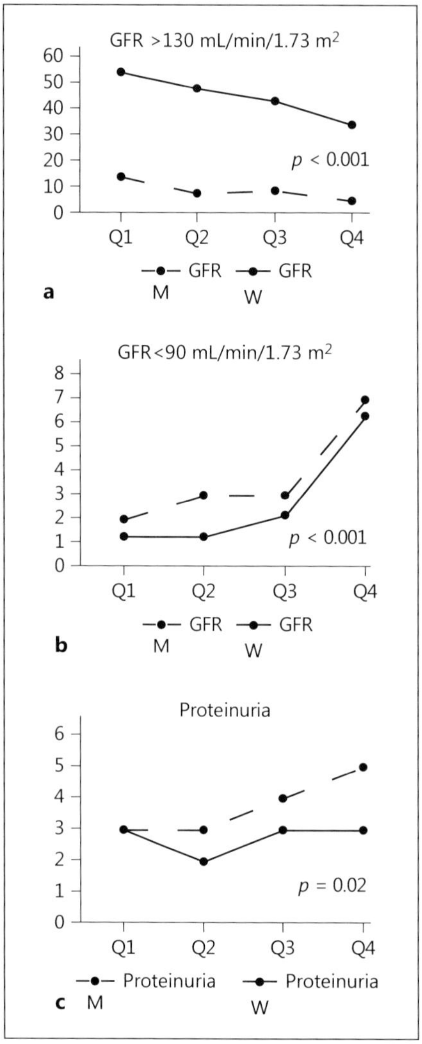

Fig. 2. a–c Relative frequency of renal function by quartiles of serum uric acid and sex. M, Men; W, women; Quartiles for uric acid (<5.3, 5.3–6.1, 6.2–6.9, ≥7 mg/dL) for men (<3.8, 3.8–4.4, 4.5–5.1 ≥5.2 mg/dL) for women linear trends of serum uric acid quartiles adjusted by sex were evaluated by Wald test, using logistic regression.

Uric Acid and Association with Impaired Renal Function

The relative frequency of subjects with GFR >130/120 mL/min/1.73 m^2 decreased as the levels uric acid increased (Fig. 2a); the frequencies of GFR <90 mL/min/1.73 m^2 were significantly higher in the Q4 of SUA (Fig. 2b); and the proteinuria was higher in M, and increased proportionally with SUA concentration (Fig. 2c).

Strength of Association and Clinical Significance of Uric Acid

Table 2 presents the association of the CRF to the SUA quartiles – CRF values were high in Q3 and Q4 of SUA. The variables that showed the greatest strength

Table 2. Association between cardiometabolic risk factors and serum uric acid (SUA) quartiles

	Q2			Q3			Q4		
	OR	95% CI	*p* value	OR	95% CI	*p* value	OR	95% CI	*p* value
Ow/Ob	1.44	1.2–1.7	<0.001	2.2	1.8–2.6	<0.001	4.1	3.4–4.9	<0.001
Hypertriglyceridemia	1.2	0.9–1.6	0.16	1.5	1.2–2.09	0.001	2.03	1.5–2.6	<0.001
LDL-c of risk	1.2	0.86–1.7	0.24	1.2	0.92–1.8	0.13	1.7	1.2–2.4	0.001
HDL-c of risk	1.1	0.9–1.3	0.22	1.18	1.006–1.4	0.04	1.4	1.2–1.7	<0.001
Hyperglycemia	1.13	0.78–1.6	0.5	1.5	1.1–2.2	0.008	1.7	1.2–2.4	0.001
Blood pressure of risk	1.06	0.57–1.9	0.85	0.85	0.46–1.5	0.85	1.1	0.65–1.9	0.63
IR	1.3	0.95–1.8	0.09	2.4	1.7–3.2	<0.001	4.7	3.5–6.3	<0.001
MetS	0.99	0.65–1.5	0.99	1.06	0.7–1.5	0.76	1.78	1.2–2.6	0.003
GFR <90 mL/min/1.73 m^2	1.07	0.6–1.9	0.8	1.2	0.7–2.1	0.46	3.2	1.9–5.4	<0.001
GFR>130/120 mL/min/1.73 m^2 M/W	0.63	0.53–0.74	<0.001	0.57	0.48–0.67	<0.001	0.39	0.32–0.46	<0.001
Proteinuria	0.77	0.47–1.2	0.31	1.1	0.74–1.8	0.5	1.3	0.83–2.08	0.24

Q, quartiles sex-specific quartiles for uric acid (<5.3, 5.3–6.1, 6.2–6.9, ≥7 mg/dL) for men (M); (<3.8, 3.8–4.4, 4.5–5.1 ≥5.2 mg/dL) for women (W). Ow/Ob, overweigh/obesity by WC and BMI; HDL-c of risk, HDL cholesterol; LDL-c of risk, LDL cholesterol; BP, blood pressure of risk; IR, insulin resistance; MetS, metabolic syndrome. OR was estimated using Q1 as a reference.

of association are located in quartile 4. This quartile was also associated with the highest probability of having CRF and with alterations of renal function such as proteinuria or lower rate of glomerular filtration.

Discussion

This epidemiological study assessing the prevalence of hyperuricemia and the strength of association between AU levels with CRF and alterations in renal function according to sex apparently included healthy young adults.

SUA levels established as risk for the development of CKD or CRF have been determined in populations with age over 30 [9, 10]. Female subjects presented lower SUA levels compared to M, which could be explained by the uricosuric effect of estrogens [15]. In this study, the overall prevalence of hyperuricemia was 16.97% (24% in M vs. 8% F), which is lower than that found by Lin [16] in a population of the same age group. In another study, Rodrigues et al. [17] reported a prevalence of high SUA concentration in adult population (25–64 years), which was similar to our results. However, they used a lower cutoff point than the one that we used (hyperuricemia M ≥6.8 M and W ≥5.4 mg/dL), suggesting that we are underestimating the real prevalence in this young population. The high prevalence of CRF in subjects with hyperuricemia is of great concern, considering that our sample consisted of young healthy adults. Notably, Kuwabara et al. [18] found that the presence of hyperuricemia alone represents a significant risk for developing cardiometabolic conditions and CKD, a risk that increases with other CRFs.

The stratification by SUA quartiles suggested that the prevalence of CRF increased significantly in Q3 (SUA levels >6.2/4.5 mg/dL M/W). Although, these concentrations of SUA are considered normal, they were significantly associated with the presence of Ow/Ob, hypertriglyceridemia, low HDL-c, hyperglycemia, and IR. In addition to the aforementioned traits, Q4 (SUA ≥7/5.2 mg/dL M/W) also included high LDL-c and MetS. Our findings are in accordance with those of previous reports that showed that excess body fat leads to increased SUA. In addition, excess visceral fat deposition increases free fatty acid release leading to higher triglyceride concentration and, increased tumor necrosis factor-alpha release and a subsequent decrease in adiponectin concentration, which finally leads to a reduction in UA renal excretion [19].

Our study showed no association between BP and SUA, presumably due to the young age of the participants. However, it is clear that relative frequency of M increased from 5% in Q3 to 12% in Q4. This finding supports a previous report from Perlstein et al. [20]. It is necessary to reiterate that in normotensive individuals, the detection of high levels of SUA may serve as an early prognostic marker to initiate preventive measures to avoid hypertension in future.

Regarding hyperglycaemia, our results concur with those reported by Wiik et al. [21], who identified that SAU levels increased the risk of developing type 2 diabetes. Hyperuricemia correlates with IR due to increased fat synthesis in liver associated with IR. There is also concurrent *de novo* purine synthesis, which accelerates uric acid production, explaining the positive association in SUA Q3 and Q4 and IR. Notably, Q3 (AU 6.2–6.9 in M and 4.5–5.1 mg/dL in W) is still considered normourecemic and is lower than those reported by Naveen and Damodar [22].

We also identified a significant increase in frequency of MetS in subjects in SUA Q4. Our findings showed an independent link between the UA and MetS levels, and this finding is consistent with that of previous studies [16, 23, 24]. Notably, such association was also found in healthy individuals [25].

Regarding renal function, SUA is an important factor associated with GFR >130/120 (M/W) mL/min/1.73 m^2. This is suggestive of probable hyperfiltration that could indicate an incipient alteration in the renal function. It has been found that the CKD-Epidemiology Collaboration formula tends to overestimate renal function [26] and to date there is no accurate cutoff point or a validated formula for its measurement in Mexicans. Q4 was strongly associated with GFR <90 mL/min/1.73 m^2. While it is not explicitly defined as CKD and cannot be considered normal GFR in young adults with no previous pathological history, this may reflect the possibility of increased risk of hyperuricemia. This may be due to decreased renal excretion of UA in the context of reduced GFR during early stages or, conversely, it could suggest that a subset of subjects with hyperuricemia can develop subtle losses in renal function. In this context, Obermayr et al. [27] reported that SUA levels between 7 and 8.9 mg/dL are associated with 1.7-fold increase in renal failure.

Our results strongly suggest that there is a strong need to establish early detection programs for CRFs and renal function assessment in young adults. In addition, we should consider reassessing the threshold levels for SUA as a risk predictor in young adults. It is well established that early diagnosis and preventive measures reduce the prevalence of CRF, which can lead to favourable cardiometabolic outcomes [28]. Hence, it is imperative to educate young adults about a healthy lifestyle and dietary recommendations to reduce the future prevalence of these known causes of morbidity and mortality.

Conclusions

High normal values of UA (≥6.2 mg/dL, for men, ≥4.5 mg/dL for women) were associated with CRF and renal impairment in young adults. It is necessary to reevaluate the appropriate cutoff points for UA in young adults, as well as to develop public health measures that allow the timely detection and treatment of this condition in this population group, thereby, reducing their long-term impact on the renal function and cardiovascular system.

References

1 Sanchez LG, Tapia E, Santamaria J, Ávila-Casado C, Soto V, Nepomuceno T, et al: Hyperuricemia induces vasoconstriction and maintains glomerular hypertension in normal and remnant kidney rats. Kidney Int 2005;67:237–247.

2 Sánchez LG, Soto V, Tapia E, et al: Role of oxidative stress in the renal abnormalities induced by experimental hyperuricemia. Am J Physiol Renal Physiol 2008;295:F1134–F1141.

3 Asakawa S, Shibata S, Morimoto C, et al: Podocyte injury and albuminuria in experimental hyperuricemic model rats. Oxid Med Cell Longev 2017;2017: 3759153.

4 Mene P, Punzoc G: Uric acid: bystander or culprit in hypertension and progressive renal disease? J Hypertens 2008;26:2085–2092.

5 Feig DI: The role of uric acid in the pathogenesis of hypertension in the young. J Clin Hypertens (Greenwich) 2012;14:346–352.

6 Filiopoulos V, Hadjiyannakos D, Vlassopoulos D: New insights into uric acid effects on the progression and prognosis of chronic kidney disease. Ren Fail 2012;34:4, 510–520.

7 Liu WC, Hung CC, Chen CS, et al: Association of hyperuricemia with renal outcomes, cardiovascular disease, and mortality. Clin J Am Soc Nephrol 2012;7:541–548.

8 Bardin T, Richette P: Definition of hyperuricemia and gouty conditions. Curr Opin Rheumatol 2014;26:186–191.

9 Desideri G, Castaldo G, Lombardi A, et al: Is it time to revise the normal range of serum uric acid levels? Eur Rev Med Pharmacol Sci 2014;18:1295–1306.

10 Kuwabara M, Bjornstada P, Hisatome I, et al: Elevated serum uric acid level predicts rapid decline in kidney function. Am J Nephrol 2017;45:330–337.
11 Leiba A, Vinker S, Dinour D, Holtzman EJ, Shani M: Uric acid levels within the normal range predict increased risk of hypertension: a cohort study. J Am Soc Hypertens 2015: 9:600–609.
12 de Miranda JA, Almeida GG, Martins RI, Cunha MB, Belo VA, dos Santos JE, Mourão-Júnior CA, Lanna CM: The role of uric acid in the insulin resistance in children and adolescents with obesity. Rev Paul Pediatr 2015; 33:431–436.
13 Alberti KG, Eckel RH, Grundy SM, Zimmet PZ, Cleeman JL, et al: Harmonizing the metabolic syndrome: a joint interim statement of the international diabetes federation task force on epidemiology and prevention; national heart, lung, and blood institute; American heart association; world heart federation; international atherosclerosis society; and international associaton for the study of obesity. Circulation 2009;120:1640–1645.
14 Kidney Disease: Improving Global Outcomes (KDIGO) CKD Work Group: KDIGO 2012 clinical practice guideline for the evaluation and management of chronic kidney disease. Kidney Int 2013;3(suppl):1–150.
15 Yadav D, Lee ES, Kim HM, Lee EY, Choi E, Chung CH: Hyperuricemia as a potential determinant of metabolic syndrome. J Lifestyle Med 2013:3:98–106.
16 Lin KP: The relationship between serum uric acid concentration and metabolic syndrome in University Freshmen. J Nurs Res 2009;17: 286–292.
17 Rodrigues SR, Baldo MP, Capingana DP, Magalhaes P, Dantas EM, et al: Distribución por género del acido urico sérico y factores de riesgo cardiovascular: estudio poblacional. Arq Bras Cardiol 2012;98:13–21.
18 Kuwabara M, Niwa K, Hisatome I, Nakagawa T, Roncal-Jimenez CA, Andres-Hernando A, Bjornstad P, et al: Asymptomatic hyperuricemia without comorbidities predicts cardiometabolic diseases: five-year Japanese cohort study. Hypertension 2017;69:1036–1044.
19 Choi HK, Mount DB, Reginato AM: Pathogenesis of gout. Ann Intern Med 2005;143: 499–516.
20 Perlstein TS, Gumieniak O, Williams GH, Sparrow D, Vokonas PS, Gaziano M, et al: Uric acid and the development of hypertension: the normative aging study. Hypertension 2006;48:1031–1036.
21 Wiik BP, Larstorp ACK, Høieggen A, Kjeldsen SE, Olsen MH, Ibsen H, et al: Serum uric acid is associated with new-onset diabetes in hypertensive patients with left ventricular hypertrophy: the LIFE study. Am J Hypertens 2010;23:845–851.
22 Naveen RA, Damodar S: Association of hyperuricemia with metabolic syndrome and insulin resistance. J Clin Diagn Res 2016; 10:OC32–OC34.
23 Onat A, Uyarel H, Hergenc G, Karabulut A, Albayrak S, Sari I, et al: Serum uric acid is a determinant of metabolic syndrome in a population-based study. Am J Hypertens 2006; 19:1055–1062.
24 Billiet L, Doaty S, Katz JD, Velasquez MT: Review of hyperuricaemia as new marker for metabolic syndrome. ISRN Rheumatol 2014; 2014:852954.
25 You L, Liu A, Wuyun G, Wu H, Wang P: Prevalence of hyperuricemia and the relationship between serum uric acid and metabolic syndrome in the Asian Mongolian area. J Arth Trombos 2014;21:355.
26 Arreola GJM, Rincón PR, Cruz RC, et al: Funcionamiento de las fórmulas MDRD-IDMS y CKD-EPI, en individuos mexicanos con función renal normal. Nefrologia 2014;34: 591–598.
27 Obermayr RP, Temml C, Gutjahr G, Knechtelsdorfer M, Oberbauer R, Klauser-Braun R: Elevated uric acid increases the risk for kidney disease. J Am Soc Nephrol 2008;19:2407–2413.
28 McMahon GM, Preis SR, Hwang SJ, et al: Mid-adulthood risk factor profiles for CKD. J Am Soc Nephrol 2014;25:2633–2641.

Monserrat Pérez-Navarro
Department of Nephrology, Hospital General de México, Dr. Eduardo Liceaga
Dr. Balmis 148 Colonia Doctores
06726 México City (México)
E-Mail lucymonsepn@yahoo.com.mx

Treviño-Becerra A, Iseki K (eds): Uric Acid in Chronic Kidney Disease.
Contrib Nephrol. Basel, Karger, 2018, vol 192, pp 135–146 (DOI: 10.1159/000484288)

Treatment of Hyperuricemia in Chronic Kidney Disease

Juan C. Ramirez-Sandoval[a] · Magdalena Madero[b]

[a]Instituto Nacional de Ciencias Médicas y Nutrición Salvador Zubirán, National Institute of Medical Sciences and Nutrition Salvador Zubirán (INCMNSZ), and [b]Instituto Nacional de Cardiología Ignacio Chávez, National Heart Institute, Mexico City, Mexico

Abstract

Hyperuricemia may be a major contributor to the development or progression of chronic kidney disease (CKD). Although there is no clear cutoff uric acid (UA) value associated to the risk for kidney damage, it appears to be an increased risk as UA rises. Lifestyle interventions such as exercise, weight reduction, low consumption of purine-rich meat, or avoiding high fructose intake are recommended for all hyperuricemic patients. Lowering urate drugs such as allopurinol or febuxostat may be an option as a renoprotective agent; yet, randomized clinical trials evaluating the safety and efficacy of these drugs are limited to a small number of single-center studies. Several ongoing clinical trials aim to evaluate the safety and efficacy of these drugs. As of today, there is insufficient evidence to recommend the widespread use of UA-lowering therapy to prevent or slow down the progression of CKD. The purpose of this review is to summarize the evidence and future perspectives about the treatment of hyperuricemia in the prevention and progression of CKD.

Introduction

Serum uric acid (SUA) levels are found to be frequently elevated in patients with chronic kidney disease (CKD). For example, in patients with predominantly nondiabetic stages 3–4 CKD, up to 66% had SUA greater than 7 mg/dL [1]. The association between SUA and CKD was historically viewed as one solely attributed to the retention of SUA caused by the glomerular filtration rate fall [2]. Nevertheless, in the last 2 decades, basic research showed that hyperuricemia plays a causal role in the progression of CKD through direct renal injury [3] and new studies suggested a possible improvement of kidney function after lowering SUA. Until today, therapeutic options as allopurinol or febuxostat for prevention of development or progression of CKD are still a matter of debate [4].

Hyperuricemia Definitions in CKD and Assessment of Risk Factors

There is great controversy about the utility of treating asymptomatic hyperuricemia either to prevent or slow down the progression of CKD, given the conflicting results in several clinical studies [5]. In addition to the issues related to methodological design and underpowered results, one of the main problems of these studies lies in the definition of hyperuricemia [6]. There are several ways to define hyperuricemia: (i) a *statistical definition* that defines hyperuricemia as SUA lying more than 2 SDs above the mean (>7.7 mg/dL in men or >6.6 mg/dL in women) [7]; (ii) a *physicochemical definition* of hyperuricemia, taking into account the saturation point for monosodium urate crystals (≥6 mg/dL) [8]; (iii) a *risk definition* based SUA values associated with an increased cardiovascular risk (8 or 9 mg/dL as the limit to begin treatment) [9] or (iv) a *risk for kidney function definition* based on upper limited expected SUA values according to serum creatinine (SCr <1.5 mg/dL: SUA >9 mg/dL, SCr 1.5–2 mg/dL: SUA >10 mg/dL, and SCr >2 mg/dL: SUA >12 mg/dL [3]).

Despite not having a clear definition of hyperuricemia, the risk between kidney damage and SUA appears to increase continuously with the level of SUA as it has been shown with hypertension and cardiovascular risk (Fig. 1) [10]. In this regard, the results of several clinical randomized trials in subjects with a mean SUA of 7 mg/dL to evaluate a short-term kidney outcome are likely to have negative results [11] compared to those studies that recruit subjects with a mean SUA of around 10 mg/dL [12].

In Figure 1, we propose a general approach in order to maximize the benefits of treating hyperuricemia to prevent or slow the progression of CKD. Given the scarce evidence, the data showed in the Figure 1 is the basis for a hypothesis that still needs to be tested in larger clinical trials. Treatment of hyperuricemia must be individualized upon evaluation of the potential benefits (prevention or avoid progression of CKD) and the risks of intervention (futility or adverse reactions).

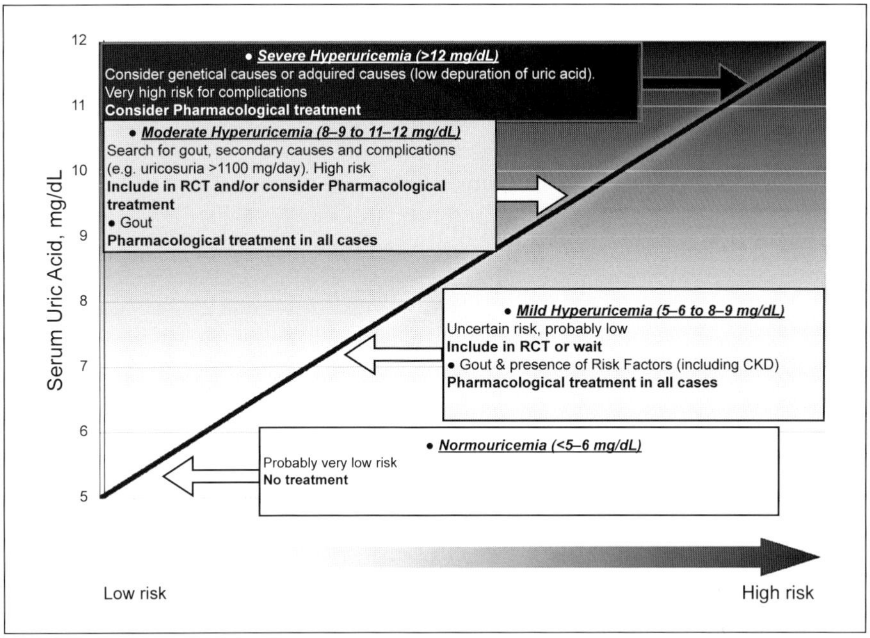

Fig. 1. Hyperuricemia and risk for kidney outcomes.

Treatment of Hyperuricemia

Lifestyle Intervention

It would be optimal that all subjects with hyperuricemia, with or without CKD, in whom treatable secondary etiologies have either been excluded or, if present, appropriately treated, could receive a specific advice with lifestyle measures in order to lower SUA. Unfortunately, there is a general lack of specific evidence from prospective, blinded, randomized clinical intervention trials that linked consumed quantities of individual dietary components to changes in SUA [13]. Most of the recommendations are taken from studies of patients with gout and are useful for treating other life-threatening comorbidities of hyperuricemic patients, including obesity, coronary artery disease, hypertension, metabolic syndrome, diabetes mellitus, and hyperlipidemia [14]. These recommendations may be summarized as follows:

1 Exercise daily and reduce weight. Weight reduction through gradual caloric restriction and exercise can help lower SUA; nevertheless, the effect of this maneuver is modest (an average weight loss of 7.7 kg over 16 weeks decrease to a mean difference of 1.6 mg/dL SUA in obese patients with gout) [15].

2 Limit consumption of purine-rich meat and seafood and consider omega-3 fatty acid supplements with regard to the evidence about higher levels of meat and seafood consumption associated with hyperuricemia [16].

3 Limit high fructose corn syrup – sweetened soft drinks and energy drinks. Fructose increases SUA given the fact that once absorbed into the cell, unregulated phosphorylation of fructose by fructokinase leads to local ATP depletion and increased AMP production [17]. Hypercaloric supplementation with fructose (+35% excess energy) at extreme doses (213–219 g/day) significantly increases SUA (mean difference = 0.5 mg/dL). Even isocaloric exchange of fructose for other carbohydrates may be useful for hypertension treatment [18]; however, this maneuver does not affect SUA in participants from 21 trials [19].

4 The consumption of low-fat or nonfat dairy products reduced consumption of saturated fat, total fat, and cholesterol has a minimal effect in lowering SUA [13].

5 Subjects must limit their intake of beer, wine, and spirits [13].

Pharmacological Treatment

Allopurinol

Allopurinol and its major active derived product, oxypurinol, inhibits the xanthine oxidase and other enzymes involved in purine and pyrimidine metabolism. Oxypurinol is a metabolite that is excreted by the kidney, and therefore, allopurinol requires dose reduction in patients with CKD [20]. One reason for caution is the accumulation of xanthine in kidney failure, which will be aggravated by the xanthine oxidase inhibitor allopurinol. Allopurinol is not a benign drug and may occasionally precipitate a hypersensitivity syndrome in 2% of patients (Stevens-Johnson-like syndrome) that can be fatal. To minimize this complication, it is recommended to initiate allopurinol at a dose of 50–100 mg/day in subjects with estimated GFR less than 30 mL/min/1.73 m^2, increasing the dose to 200 or 300 mg/day every 2–5 weeks to achieve desired UA levels of <6 mg/dL; doses >300 mg/day are permitted so long as they are accompanied by appropriate patient education and monitoring for toxicity (e.g., pruritus, rash, elevated hepatic transaminases) [13]. Adherence to these published allopurinol dosing guidelines led to suboptimal control of hyperuricemia in most patients [21].

Febuxostat

The newer xanthine oxidase inhibitor, febuxostat, is a non-purine urate-lowering drug with more efficiency and specificity for the reduced and oxidized forms of xanthine oxidase than allopurinol [22]. Febuxostat is metabolized mainly by the liver, has its elimination is primarily through renal and biliary routes, is effective and well tolerated in patients with mild CKD, and appears to be less frequently associated with hypersensitivity or nephrotoxicity; yet the most commonly reported

Table 1. Drugs that may affect SUA

Drug	Mechanism	Evidence	Comment
Topiroxostat	Xanthine oxidase inhibitor	Reduce 45 SUA and 33% the levels of albuminuria [36]	Profile similar to febuxostat
Benzbromarone	Uricosuric	In CKD subjects, kidney function did not improve by reducing the SUA levels with benzbromarone [37]	Potentially hepatotoxic
Losartan	Unique angiotensin receptor blocker which blockade URAT 1 (uricosuric)	In posthoc analysis of REENAL, the risk of doubling of SCr or development of CKD 5 was decreased by 6% for every 0.5 mg/dL decrement in SUA [38]	Uricosuric effect of losartan accounts for approximately one-fifth of its renoprotective effects
Acetylsalicylic acid	High dosages (>3 gm/day) are uricosuric, while low dosages (75–325 mg/day) cause SUA retention	Increase SUA and rates of acute gout flares in patients with prevalent gout and cardiovascular prophylaxis	Discontinuation is generally not required, given the beneficial effects on mortality [13]
SGLT2 inhibitors	Uricosuric	In subjects with diabetes, reduce SUA by 0.3–0.9 mg/dL [39]	Small SUA reductions alone unlikely explain the observed renal and cardiovascular benefits
Fenofibrate	Uricosuric	200 mg/day reduced a 19% in SUA	
Vitamin C	Uricosuric	Supplementation with 500 mg/day of vitamin C for 2 months reduces SUA [40]	May induce hyperoxaluria

* SGLT2 inhibitors, sodium glucose co-transporter 2; CKD, chronic kidney disease; SUA, serum uric acid.

adverse drug reactions are liver function abnormalities, diarrhea, and rash [23]. For example, in the CONFIRMS trial with 2,269 subjects with gout, febuxostat 40 mg, febuxostat 80 mg, or allopurinol 300 mg (200 mg in subjects with CKD3) reduced SUA less than 6 mg/dL in 45, 67, and 42% of patients respectively [24].

Other drugs with beneficial effect on hyperuricemia are shown in Table 1.

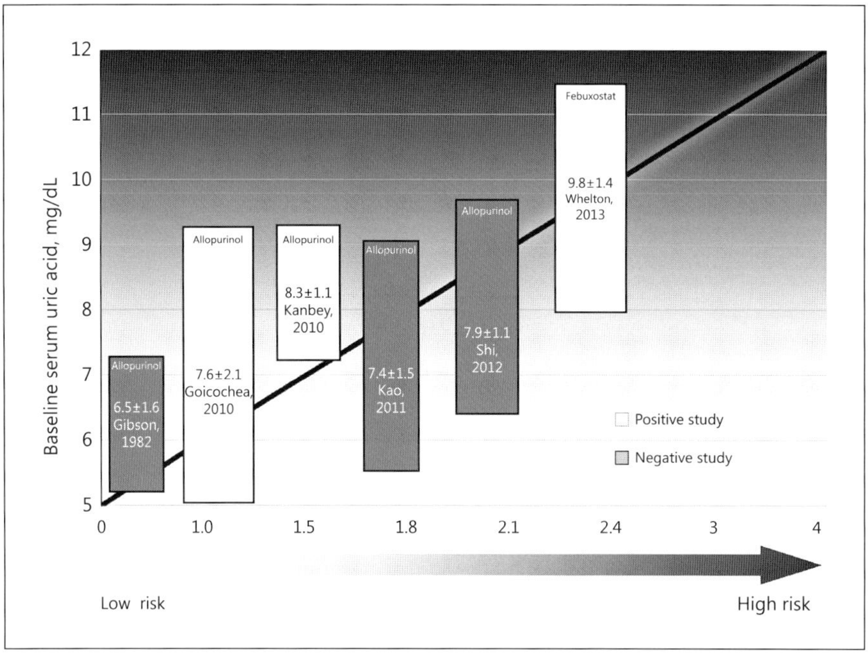

Fig. 2. Baseline hyperuricemia in trials with urate-lowering drugs using change in eGFR as outcome. Clinical trials, which showed a positive effect in eGFR of urate-lowering drugs, are in the white box and those with a negative or inconclusive result are in the gray box.

Alopurinol Treatment and Kidney Outcomes

The available evidence from randomized clinical trials (RCT) is scarce in terms of a small number of single-center trials, variable duration of follow-up, and clinical heterogeneity in trials evaluating baseline kidney function and proteinuria.

A systematic review of 8 randomized controlled trials (n = 476) [11] was performed to evaluate the benefits and risks of UA-lowering therapy with allopurinol compared with placebo. According to these studies, even allopurinol decreased SUA (mean difference of –2.5 mg/dL, 95% CI from –3.3 to –1.7 mg/dL, $p < 0.001$), in 5 RCTs (n = 346, Fig. 2); these studies also reported estimated glomerular filtration rate (eGFR). There was no significant difference in the change in eGFR from baseline between the allopurinol and control arms (mean difference of 3.1 mL/min/1.73 m^2, 95% CI from –0.9 to 7.1 mL/min/1.73 m^2, $p = 0.1$) [12, 25–28]. The remaining 3 trials (n = 130) reporting only creatinine data showed that the change in SCr concentration from baseline was in favor of allopurinol (mean difference –0.4 mg/dL, 95% CI from –0.8 to –0.0

mg/dL, $p = 0.03$). In this meta-analysis, there were not significant differences with respect the changes in proteinuria or blood pressure, and it was not possible to analyze progression of CKD in the wake of scarce and heterogeneity of data.

In another meta-analysis of 19 RCTs enrolling 992 patients with stage 3–5 CKD, allopurinol significantly reduced SUA levels, blood pressure, and a small but potentially clinically important and statistically significant improvement in eGFR was noted with a mean difference of 3.2 mL/min/1.73 m^2 (95% CI from 0.16 to –6.2 mL/min/1.73 m^2, $p = 0.039$) [29].

Using a different approach, after a group of investigators withdrew allopurinol from subjects with stable CKD, there was an acceleration of eGFR loss in the patients who were not taking angiotensin-converting-enzyme inhibitors [30].

Febuxostat Treatment and Kidney Outcomes

Approximately 30–40% of patients with gout have some degree of kidney impairment [31]. In the open-label clinical trial, 113 subjects with gout and baseline SUA of 9.7 ± 1.3 mg/dL received febuxostat for 5 years: subjects initially received febuxostat 80 mg/day; between weeks 4 and 24, the dose could be titrated to 40 or 120 mg/day to maintain an SUA between less than 6.0 mg/dL but not lower than 3.0 mg/dL. Those with the greatest reductions in SUA experienced reduced rates of kidney deterioration or even stabilization of kidney function. For every 1 mg/dL decrease in SUA, the model projected an expected improvement in eGFR of 1 mL/min from the untreated value [32].

In the Febuxostat/Allopurinol Comparative Extension Long-term Study, 1,086 subjects with a mean SUA level of 9.8 mg/dL were treated with febuxostat 80 or 120 mg daily, or allopurinol 300 mg daily. The use of febuxostat was shown to preserve kidney function. Greater continued reductions in SUA levels were reported to be associated with less decline in kidney function. For every 1 mg/dL of long-term reduction in SUA, 1.2 mL/min/1.73 m^2 of eGFR would be preserved [12].

In another single-center study, febuxostat, 40 mg, once daily for 6 months, was compared with placebo in subjects with CKD stages 3 and 4, with asymptomatic hyperuricemia. Mean eGFR in the febuxostat group showed a nonsignificant increase from 31.5 ± 13 to 33.7 ± 16.6 mL/min/1.73 m^2 at 6 months. With placebo, the mean eGFR decreased from a baseline of 32.6 ± 11.6–28.2 ± 11.5 mL/min/1.73 m^2 ($p = 0.003$) [33].

Table 2. Ongoing randomized clinical trials

Randomized	Name	Objective	Population
CKD-FIX study [41]	The Controlled trial of slowing of kidney disease progression From the Inhibition of Xanthine oxidase	To assess the effect of allopurinol on slowing the decline of eGFR	620 patients with stages 3–4 CKD
FEATHER [42]	Febuxostat versus placebo randomized controlled trial regarding reduced renal function in patients with hyperuricemia complicated by CKD stage 3	To assess the effect of allopurinol versus placebo on slowing the decline of eGFR	400 Japanese patients aged 20 or older who have hyperuricemia without gouty arthritis, who present with CKD stage 3, and whose SUA concentration is 7.1–10.0 mg/dL
The PERL [43]	The preventing early renal loss	To assess the effect of allopurinol (dose ranging 200–400 mg) or placebo on the GFR following the 3-year treatment period, measured by the plasma clearance of non-radioactive iohexol (iGFR) and adjusted for the iGFR at baseline	Clinical trial at 8 diabetes centers, enrolling approximately 480 patients with type 1 diabetes who are at increased risk of developing kidney disease
Other RCT	Febuxostat and benzbromarone [44]	To assess the effect of febuxostat and benzbromarone for changes in proteinuria and eGFR	CKD patients With GFR 20–50 mL/min
	Verinurad and febuxostat [45]	To assess the potential clinical benefits of the combination of Verinurad, a novel Urate Transporter 1 inhibitor, and Febuxostat in lowering concentrations of circulating uric acid and thus improving kidney or cardiovascular status of	Patients with hyperuricemia, albuminuria, and type 2 diabetes

CKD, chronic kidney disease; eGFR, estimated glomerular filtration rate; SUA, serum uric acid; RCT, randomized clinical trials.

Ongoing Trials

The inconclusive evidence with regard to urate-lowering treatment and the urgent need for new and effective treatments to prevent or slow progression of CKD has to be further investigated and large-scale RCT has been planned (Table 2).

Controversies

There is lack of knowledge if the beneficial effect of allopurinol is due to the reduction of SUA or to a reduction in xanthine oxidase-associated oxidants [17].

Although SUA may have proinflammatory effects on vascular cells and adipocytes, it can also function as an antioxidant [34].

Positive studies of febuxostat in patients with gout may not be generalized to those with asymptomatic hyperuricemia, since gout patients have a different risk phenotype. Furthermore, the mechanism of kidney protection related to febuxostat may be associated with a low use of NSAIDS given a lower number of acute flairs, and not related to lowering SUA [35].

Conclusions

Despite the unclear evidence that links SUA value to the risk for kidney damage, it appears as if the risk increases continuously with the level of serum urate. Lifestyle interventions such as exercise, weight reduction, low consumption of purine-rich meat, or avoiding high fructose intake are recommended for all hyperuricemic patients although the efficacy of these interventions is modest. Lowering urate drugs such as allopurinol or febuxostat may be an option as a renoprotective agent; yet RCT evidence evaluating the safety and efficacy of these drugs are limited to a small number of single-center studies with suboptimal methodology. Standarized definitions of hyperuricemia in clinical trials that include high-risk patients would probably yield more definitive results.

References

1 Madero M, Sarnak MJ, Wang X, Greene T, Beck GJ, Kusek JW, et al: Uric acid and long-term outcomes in CKD. Am J Kidney Dis 2009;53:796–803.

2 Johnson RJ, Nakagawa T, Jalal D, Sánchez-Lozada LG, Kang DH, Ritz E: Uric acid and chronic kidney disease: which is chasing which? Nephrol Dial Transplant 2013;28: 2221–2228.

3 Johnson RJ, Kivlighn SD, Kim YG, Suga S, Fogo AB: Reappraisal of the pathogenesis and consequences of hyperuricemia in hypertension, cardiovascular disease, and renal disease. Am J Kidney Dis 1999;33:225–234.

4 Eleftheriadis T, Golphinopoulos S, Pissas G, Stefanidis I: Asymptomatic hyperuricemia and chronic kidney disease: narrative review of a treatment controversial. J Adv Res 2017; 8:555–560.

5 Kumagai T, Ota T, Tamura Y, Chang WX, Shibata S, Uchida S: Time to target uric acid to retard CKD progression. Clin Exp Nephrol 2017;21:182–192.
6 Borghi C, Rosei EA, Bardin T, Dawson J, Dominiczak A, Kielstein JT, et al: Serum uric acid and the risk of cardiovascular and renal disease. J Hypertens 2015;33:1729–1741.
7 Chen JH, Yeh WT, Chuang SY, Wu YY, Pan WH: Gender-specific risk factors for incident gout: a prospective cohort study. Clin Rheumatol 2012;31:239–245.
8 Loeb JN: The influence of temperature on the solubility of monosodium urate. Arthritis Rheum 1972;15:189–192.
9 Yamanaka H: Japanese Society of Gout and Nucleic Acid Metabolism: Japanese guideline for the management of hyperuricemia and gout: second edition. Nucleosides Nucleotides Nucleic Acids 2011;30:1018–1029.
10 Grayson PC, Kim SY, LaValley M, Choi HK: Hyperuricemia and incident hypertension: a systematic review and meta-analysis. Arthritis Care Res 2011;63:102–110.
11 Bose B, Badve SV, Hiremath SS, Boudville N, Brown FG, Cass A, et al: Effects of uric acid-lowering therapy on renal outcomes: a systematic review and meta-analysis. Nephrol Dial Transplant 2014;29:406–413.
12 Whelton A, MacDonald PA, Chefo S, Gunawardhana L: Preservation of renal function during gout treatment with febuxostat: a quantitative study. Postgrad Med 2013;125: 106–114.
13 Khanna D, Fitzgerald JD, Khanna PP, Bae S, Singh MK, Neogi T, et al: American college of rheumatology guidelines for management of gout. Part 1: systematic nonpharmacologic and pharmacologic therapeutic approaches to hyperuricemia. Arthritis Care Res 2012;64: 1431–1446.
14 Choi HK: A prescription for lifestyle change in patients with hyperuricemia and gout. Curr Opin Rheumatol 2010;22:165–172.
15 Dessein PH, Shipton EA, Stanwix AE, Joffe BI, Ramokgadi J: Beneficial effects of weight loss associated with moderate calorie/carbohydrate restriction, and increased proportional intake of protein and unsaturated fat on serum urate and lipoprotein levels in gout: a pilot study. Ann Rheum Dis 2000;59:539–543.
16 Lim JH, Kim Y, Kim Y, Na S, Rhee M, Lee M: Relationship between serum uric acid levels, metabolic syndrome, and arterial stiffness in Korean. Korean Circ J 2010;40:314–320.
17 Johnson RJ, Sautin YY, Oliver WJ, Roncal C, Mu W, Gabriela Sanchez-Lozada L, et al: Lessons from comparative physiology: could uric acid represent a physiologic alarm signal gone awry in western society? J Comp Physiol 2009;179:67–76.
18 Madero M, Rodriguez Castellanos FE, Jalal D, Villalobos-Martin M, Salazar J, Vazquez-Rangel A, et al: A pilot study on the impact of a low fructose diet and allopurinol on clinic blood pressure among overweight and prehypertensive subjects: a randomized placebo controlled trial. J Am Soc Hypertens 2015;9: 837–844.
19 Zhao CC, Wang AP, Li LX, Li TT, Chen MY, Zhu Y, et al: Urine uric acid excretion is associated with nonalcoholic fatty liver disease in patients with type 2 diabetes. J Diabetes Complications 2016;30:1074–1080.
20 Zhang W, Doherty M, Bardin T, Pascual E, Barskova V, Conaghan P, et al: EULAR evidence based recommendations for gout. Part II: management. Report of a task force of the EULAR Standing Committee For International Clinical Studies Including Therapeutics (ESCISIT). Ann Rheum Dis 2006;65: 1312–1324.
21 Dalbeth N, Stamp LK: Gout: why compare the effectiveness of suboptimal gout management? Nat Rev Rheumatol 2015;11:506–507.
22 Takano Y, Hase-Aoki K, Horiuchi H, Zhao L, Kasahara Y, Kondo S, et al: Selectivity of febuxostat, a novel non-purine inhibitor of xanthine oxidase/xanthine dehydrogenase. Life Sci 2005;76:1835–1847.
23 Grabowski BA, Khosravan R, Vernillet L, Mulford DJ: Metabolism and excretion of [14C] febuxostat, a novel nonpurine selective inhibitor of xanthine oxidase, in healthy male subjects. J Clin Pharmacol 2011;51:189–201.
24 Becker MA, Schumacher HR, Espinoza LR, Wells AF, MacDonald P, Lloyd E, et al: The urate-lowering efficacy and safety of febuxostat in the treatment of the hyperuricemia of gout: the CONFIRMS trial. Arthritis Res Ther 2010;12:R63.

25 Goicoechea M, de Vinuesa SG, Verdalles U, Ruiz-Caro C, Ampuero J, Rincón A, et al: Effect of allopurinol in chronic kidney disease progression and cardiovascular risk. Clin J Am Soc Nephrol 2010;5:1388–1393.
26 Kanbay M, Jensen T, Solak Y, Le M, Roncal-Jimenez C, Rivard C, et al: Uric acid in metabolic syndrome: from an innocent bystander to a central player. Eur J Intern Med 2016;29: 3–8.
27 Kao MP, Ang DS, Gandy SJ, Nadir MA, Houston JG, Lang CC, et al: Allopurinol benefits left ventricular mass and endothelial dysfunction in chronic kidney disease. J Am Soc Nephrol 2011;22:1382–1389.
28 Shi Y, Chen W, Jalal D, Li Z, Chen W, Mao H, et al: Clinical outcome of hyperuricemia in IgA nephropathy: a retrospective cohort study and randomized controlled trial. Kidney Blood Press Res 2012;35:153–160.
29 Kanji T, Gandhi M, Clase CM, Yang R: Urate lowering therapy to improve renal outcomes in patients with chronic kidney disease: systematic review and meta-analysis. BMC Nephrol 2015;16:58.
30 Talaat KM, El-Sheikh AR: The effect of mild hyperuricemia on urinary transforming growth factor beta and the progression of chronic kidney disease. Am J Nephrol 2007; 27:435–440.
31 Juraschek SP, Kovell LC, Miller ER 3rd, Gelber AC, Hopkins J: Gout, urate lowering therapy and uric acid levels among US adults HHS public access. Arthritis Care Res 2015; 67:588–592.
32 Whelton A, Macdonald PA, Zhao L, Hunt B, Gunawardhana L: Renal function in gout: long-term treatment effects of febuxostat. J Clin Rheumatol 2011;17:7–13.
33 Sircar D, Chatterjee S, Waikhom R, Golay V, Raychaudhury A, Chatterjee S, et al: Efficacy of febuxostat for slowing the GFR decline in patients with CKD and asymptomatic hyperuricemia: a 6-month, double-blind, randomized, placebo-controlled trial. Am J Kidney Dis 2015;66:945–950.
34 Sánchez-Lozada LG, Soto V, Tapia E, Avila-Casado C, Sautin YY, Nakagawa T, et al: Role of oxidative stress in the renal abnormalities induced by experimental hyperuricemia. Am J Physiol Renal Physiol 2008;295:F1134–F1141.
35 Schumacher HR Jr, Becker MA, Lloyd E, MacDonald PA, Lademacher C: Febuxostat in the treatment of gout: 5-years findings of the FOCUS efficacy and safety study. Rheumatology 2009;48:188–194.
36 Hosoya T, Ohno I, Nomura S, Hisatome I, Uchida S, Fujimori S, et al: Effects of topiroxostat on the serum urate levels and urinary albumin excretion in hyperuricemic stage 3 chronic kidney disease patients with or without gout. Clin Exp Nephrol. 2014;18:876–884.
37 Fujimori S, Ooyama K, Ooyama H, Moromizato H: Efficacy of benzbromarone in hyperuricemic patients associated with chronic kidney disease. Nucleosides Nucleotides Nucleic Acids 2011;30:1035–1038.
38 Miao Y, Ottenbros SA, Laverman GD, Brenner BM, Cooper ME, Parving HH, et al: Effect of a reduction in uric acid on renal outcomes during losartan treatment: a post hoc analysis of the reduction of endpoints in non-insulin-dependent diabetes mellitus with the angiotensin II antagonist losartan trial. Hypertension 2011;58:2–7.
39 Van Bommel EJ, Muskiet MH, Tonneijck L, Kramer MH, Nieuwdorp M, Van Raalte DH: In-depth review SGLT2 inhibition in the diabetic kidney-from mechanisms to clinical outcome. Clin J Am Soc Nephrol 2016;12: 700–710.
40 Huang HY, Appel LJ, Choi MJ, Gelber AC, Charleston J, Norkus EP, et al: The effects of vitamin C supplementation on serum concentrations of uric acid: results of a randomized controlled trial. Arthritis Rheum 2005; 52:1843–1847.
41 National Research Infrastructure for Australia: Trial Review – ANZCTR, 2016. https://www.anzctr.org.au/Trial/Registration/TrialReview.aspx?ACTRN=12613000513718.
42 Hosoya T, Kimura K, Itoh S, Inaba M, Uchida S, Tomino Y, et al: The effect of febuxostat to prevent a further reduction in renal function of patients with hyperuricemia who have never had gout and are complicated by chronic kidney disease stage 3: study protocol for a multicenter randomized controlled study. Trials 2014;15:26.

43 Maahs DM, Caramori L, Cherney DZ, Galecki AT, Gao C, Jalal D, et al: Uric acid lowering to prevent kidney function loss in diabetes: the preventing early renal function loss (PERL) allopurinol study. Curr Diab Rep 2013;13:550–559.
44 Ling W: Compare the Renal Protective Effects of Febuxostat and Benzbromarone – Tabular View – ClinicalTrials.gov [Internet]. https://clinicaltrials.gov/ct2/show/record/NCT02338323?term=febuxostat&recrs=a&rank=3 (cited July 29, 2017).
45 AstraZeneca. Intensive Uric Acid Lowering With RDEA3170 and Febuxostat in Patients With Albuminuria – Tabular View – ClinicalTrials.gov [Internet]. https://clinicaltrials.gov/ct2/show/record/NCT03118739?term=febuxostat&recrs=a&rank=4 (cited Jul 29, 2017).

Magdalena Madero
Instituto Nacional de Cardiología Ignacio Chávez, National Heart Institute
Juan Badiano 1 Col. Sección XVI
Tlalpan, CDMX, 14080, México City (Mexico)
E-Mail madero.magdalena@gmail.com

Author Index

Subject Index